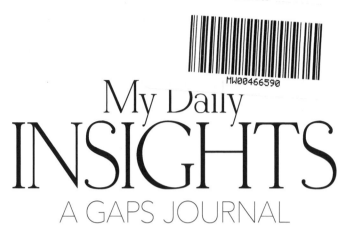

My Daily
INSIGHTS
A GAPS JOURNAL

Cover and interior design: Liz Mrofka
Cover image: Supatida Suriyachan
Copy editing and proofing: Amy Mihaly
Printing: CreateSpace

Be Well Press
5803 McWhinney Blvd.
Loveland, CO 80538
BeWellClinic.net

ISBN-13: 978-0-9983300-2-0
ISBN-10: 0-9983300-2-7

My Daily
INSIGHTS
A GAPS JOURNAL

Amy Mihaly, FNP-BC, CGP

Introduction

Welcome! You hold in your hands a helpful tool. But having a tool is not enough—you need to know what it's for and how to use it! The following pages explain why this tool was created, and how it's designed to be used. But remember, a tool is absolutely worthless on the shelf, so keep this out and use it every day!

I have followed the GAPS protocol for years, and I know how hard it is. You are supposed to remember what you ate that day and how it made you feel. Each day there are numerous supplements and foods to keep track of. And in the midst of all this remembering you are supposed to prepare your food, rest, think positive thoughts and still complete your responsibilities in job and household! This is a tall order, and one of the primary reasons why many people are not successful on the GAPS protocol.

Only you can prepare food and make your schedule, but what if you had a tool that assisted you with other things? What if this tool reminded you of daily habits, provided a place to track your symptoms and meals, and prompted you to refresh your mind?

This is what *My Daily Insights: A GAPS Journal* is designed to do. Each page gives you quick reminders about the things you should do every day, and a place to track them. A quote and journaling prompt are provided for a short yet important focus on your mindsets and emotions. I believe that one reason for my success in healing has been my determination to fight for hope, to choose gratitude, and to care about others. To me, this is as important as any food or supplements I have taken. Fighting for this attitude is a regular battle, and I hope that the inclusion of these quotes can help you win it often.

I want this to be a helpful tool, and I need your help. Nothing can be perfect or exactly personalized, but please feel free to share any feedback that you have. I wish you strength and success on this journey! Onward!

—*Amy Mihaly*

How to Use This Journal

- This is meant to be a quick check in. Spend only 5-10 minutes on it. It's designed to be efficient so you will actually do it!

- Consider using your journal morning and evening.

  - ❖ In the morning read the quote, and journal to set your mood for the day. Then, from the checklist at the top remind yourself of your daily habits and make a plan of how you will complete them.

  - ❖ In the evening, record your intake, symptoms, and other relevant thoughts or notes before going to bed.

  - ❖ Optionally, keep the journal nearby to record your meals and check off daily habits as you do them.

- Keep going, even if you miss a day. Your goal is to record the big picture. If you miss a day here and there, you still have a good representation of your health journey. Don't let a small failure throw you off. No matter how many days you have missed, pick up where you left off and keep going!

- Once a week a little more time is required to fill out the Week-At-A-Glance page. This is a one-page summary of the previous week. Plan for this to take 10-15 minutes.

  - ❖ This page gives the quickest summary to you and/or your practitioner. Make sure to fill this in, no matter how many daily pages you filled in the previous week.

- A quote and journal prompt are published daily on our blog at www.notesandinsights.com, where comments are encouraged. You can subscribe to receive this encouragement in your inbox daily.

- This is your tool, so use it in whatever way works best for you!

Example: Daily Page

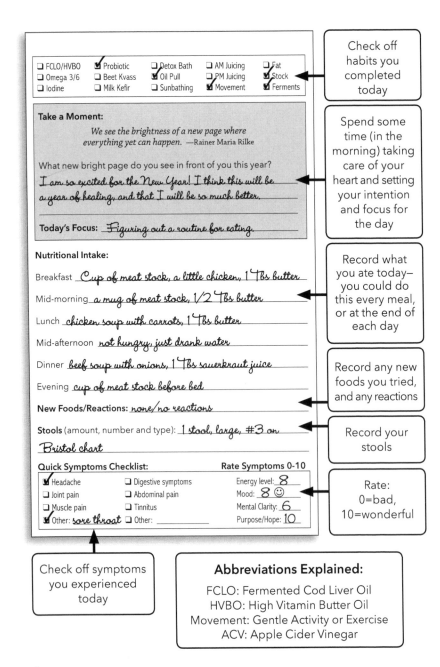

❏ FCLO/HVBO ☑ Probiotic ❏ Detox Bath ❏ AM Juicing ❏ Fat
❏ Omega 3/6 ❏ Beet Kvass ☑ Oil Pull ❏ PM Juicing ☑ Stock
❏ Iodine ❏ Milk Kefir ❏ Sunbathing ☑ Movement ☑ Ferments

Take a Moment:

We see the brightness of a new page where
everything yet can happen. —Rainer Maria Rilke

What new bright page do you see in front of you this year?
I am so excited for the New Year! I think this will be
a year of healing, and that I will be so much better.

Today's Focus: *Figuring out a routine for eating.*

Nutritional Intake:

Breakfast *Cup of meat stock, a little chicken, 1 Tbs butter*

Mid-morning *a mug of meat stock, 1/2 Tbs butter*

Lunch *chicken soup with carrots, 1 Tbs butter*

Mid-afternoon *not hungry, just drank water*

Dinner *beef soup with onions, 1 Tbs sauerkraut juice*

Evening *cup of meat stock before bed*

New Foods/Reactions: *none/no reactions*

Stools (amount, number and type): *1 stool, large, #3 on*
Bristol chart

Quick Symptoms Checklist: **Rate Symptoms 0-10**

☑ Headache   ❏ Digestive symptoms   Energy level: *8*
❏ Joint pain   ❏ Abdominal pain   Mood: *8* ☺
❏ Muscle pain   ❏ Tinnitus   Mental Clarity: *6*
☑ Other: *sore throat* ❏ Other: _____   Purpose/Hope: *10*

Check off habits you completed today

Spend some time (in the morning) taking care of your heart and setting your intention and focus for the day

Record what you ate today— you could do this every meal, or at the end of each day

Record any new foods you tried, and any reactions

Record your stools

Rate: 0=bad, 10=wonderful

Check off symptoms you experienced today

Abbreviations Explained:

FCLO: Fermented Cod Liver Oil
HVBO: High Vitamin Butter Oil
Movement: Gentle Activity or Exercise
ACV: Apple Cider Vinegar

Example: Week-At-A-Glance

Week-At-A-Glance

My week overall: 0----------------------------|--------------------10

I would describe my week (in one word) as: __ready__

Because? __I feel more prepared for this try on GAPS__

General progress:

Advanced to a new stage? (Y)/N   Current stage? __Stage 2__

New foods tolerated: __egg yolks__ Foods removed: _____

Animal fats consumed: __butter, lard__ Avg. daily amount: __1/2 cup__

# of days stock consumed: __7__   Avg. daily amount: __2 cups__

Probiotics/fermented foods/cultured dairy:

Probiotic supplement: __Bio-Kult__ Current dose: __1/4 capsule__

Die-off symptoms (Y)/N   Describe: __headache, sore throat__

_____

Beet Kvass __1 Tbs__   Sour Cream __1 Tsp__

Veggie Medley __1 Tsp__   Yogurt __none__

Sauerkraut __1 Tsp juice__   Kefir __none__

Detoxing Progress: (Apple Cider Vinegar)

# of detox baths: __6__   Ingredients: (ACV)/(Epsom)/Baking soda

# of days sunbathed: __2__ # of minutes per session: __5__ minutes

# of days juiced in am: __0__ _____ in pm: __0__

Ingredients: __n/a__

Overall reactions to detoxing: __sore throat, HA-detox bath helped__

Symptoms descriptions:

Stools: Daily Y/(N)   #per day __0-1__   Type(s): #2-#4 (Bristol)

Digestion: __upset stomach first day, tried egg yolks__

Mood/energy: __good energy the first 3 days, now more tired__

Memory/clarity: __average for me, poor memory__

Sleep/Stress: __sleeping well__

Typical-for-me symptoms: __headache almost every day, very tired__

Overall rating of your week

Details about stages, overall progress, and food amounts

Details about probiotics, ferments, and any die-off reactions

Overall picture of how detoxing went this week

Description of symptoms, you can also rate them as better, same or worse

Describe other symptoms, including your typical ones

Finding Your Why

When you start something new, excitement and motivation are usually high, but those feelings can disappear when things get difficult or monotonous.

To combat this, remind yourself of your why—why you started doing this and why it's important to you. So take time now, when your reasons are clear, to write down why you want to be on this journey. Then come back to it as you need to. Here are some questions to help you get started.

What is it that you want? What do you want to stop? What do you care about? Why is it worth it? What will be better?

I want to line my life up fears!
I want to stop second guessing due to fear
and anxiety.
I care about my health, & family.
I get to truly live!
My life will be much better.

Now, combine those thoughts in an easy-to-remember statement. Write your own statement following the example below. Then copy it and put it somewhere you can see everyday.

Example:
I am (doing GAPS diet, not eating junk food, removing chemical products) because I want to (be free of headaches, live long enough to meet my grandchildren, be able to go back to work).

My Why: *I'm doing Gaps diet because I*
want to actually live life!

New Beginnings

*No matter how short or long
your journey to your accomplishment is,
if you don't begin you can't get there.
Beginning is difficult, but unavoidable!*

—Israelmore Ayivor

172 lbs.

Date June 9, 2022

- ❏ FCLO/HVBO
- ☑ Probiotic
- ❏ Detox Bath
- ❏ AM Juicing
- ☑ Fat
- ❏ Omega 3/6
- ❏ Beet Kvass
- ❏ Oil Pull
- ❏ PM Juicing
- ❏ Stock
- ❏ Iodine
- ❏ Milk Kefir
- ❏ Sunbathing
- ❏ Movement
- ❏ Ferments

Take a Moment:

We see the brightness of a new page where everything yet can happen. —Rainer Maria Rilke

What new bright page do you see in front of you this year?

I see overall health.

Today's Focus: Lots of soup and afternoon fast.

Nutritional Intake:

Breakfast Chicken Soup & coffee

Mid-morning Ginger tea (nausea)

Lunch Chicken soup

Mid-afternoon

Dinner Electrolytes

Evening "

New Foods/Reactions:

Stools (amount, number and type): 1 - # 6 on Bristol chart.

Quick Symptoms Checklist: **Rate Symptoms 0-10**

- ☑ Headache
- ☑ Digestive symptoms Reflux
- ❏ Joint pain
- ❏ Abdominal pain
- ❏ Muscle pain
- ❏ Tinnitus
- ☑ Other: tired
- ❏ Other:

Energy level: 4
Mood: 8
Mental Clarity: 4
Purpose/Hope: 10

10

Date June 10, 2022

❏ FCLO/HVBO	❏ Probiotic	❏ Detox Bath	❏ AM Juicing	☑ Fat
❏ Omega 3/6	❏ Beet Kvass	❏ Oil Pull	❏ PM Juicing	❏ Stock
❏ Iodine	❏ Milk Kefir	❏ Sunbathing	❏ Movement	☑ Ferments

Take a Moment:

> *Life is not easy for any of us. But what of that?*
> *We must have perseverance and above all confidence in ourselves.*
> *We must believe that we are gifted for something, and that this thing,*
> *at whatever cost, must be attained.* —Marie Curie

What do you feel like you were gifted to pursue?

Health and knowledge of health. This experience is opening a new world!

Today's Focus: Get more fats and organs.

Nutritional Intake:

Breakfast Chicken soup & coffee

Mid-morning

Lunch Chicken soup w/ pumpkin puree, duck fat
2 eggs

Mid-afternoon

Dinner Fasting - Electrolytes

Evening

New Foods/Reactions:

Stools (amount, number and type): 1 # 1 on the Bristol Scale

Quick Symptoms Checklist: Rate Symptoms 0-10

☑ Headache	❏ Digestive symptoms	Energy level: 5
❏ Joint pain	❏ Abdominal pain	Mood: 8
❏ Muscle pain	❏ Tinnitus	Mental Clarity: 4
❏ Other:	☑ Other: Heart burn	Purpose/Hope: 10

11

Date June 11, 2022

☐ FCLO/HVBO	☐ Probiotic	☐ Detox Bath	☐ AM Juicing	☒ Fat
☒ Omega 3/6	☐ Beet Kvass	☐ Oil Pull	☐ PM Juicing	☒ Stock
☐ Iodine	☐ Milk Kefir	☐ Sunbathing	☐ Movement	☒ Ferments

Take a Moment:

Start by doing what's necessary, then what's possible, and suddenly you are doing the impossible. — St. Francis of Assisi

Think about approaching your health like this. What can you start with that is necessary?

Stay compliant. Take it one meal at a time.

Today's Focus: Feel up.

Nutritional Intake:

Breakfast Chicken soup w/ pumpkin puree. 1 egg. Coffee +

Mid-morning Avocado w/ sert rox & soup

Lunch Chicken soup w/ pumpkin puree. Scallops Avocado w/ chimichurri sauce.

Mid-afternoon

Dinner Salmon & scallops w/ chimichurri sauce.

Evening

New Foods/Reactions: Salmon, scallops, sauce & Avocado. Diarrhea @ night.

Stools (amount, number and type): #5 & #7

Quick Symptoms Checklist: Rate Symptoms 0-10

☐ Headache	☒ Digestive symptoms	Energy level: 4
☐ Joint pain	☒ Abdominal pain	Mood: 10
☐ Muscle pain	☐ Tinnitus	Mental Clarity: 6
☐ Other:	☐ Other:	Purpose/Hope: 10

12

Date June 12, 2022

- [ ] FCLO/HVBO
- [ ] Omega 3/6
- [ ] Iodine
- [ ] Probiotic
- [ ] Beet Kvass
- [ ] Milk Kefir
- [ ] Detox Bath
- [ ] Oil Pull
- [x] Sunbathing
- [ ] AM Juicing
- [ ] PM Juicing
- [ ] Movement
- [x] Fat
- [x] Stock
- [x] Ferments

Take a Moment:

Human beings, by changing the inner attitudes of their minds, can change the outer aspects of their lives. —Willam James

What mind attitudes do you need to change to succeed?

To just do it.

Today's Focus: Making sure Im set up to succeed this week.

Nutritional Intake:

Breakfast Avocado, saurkraut, 2 Eggs. Cofee w/ collagen. a no pods.

Mid-morning

Lunch Deer stew w/ liver

Mid-afternoon

Dinner

Evening

New Foods/Reactions:

Stools (amount, number and type): None

Quick Symptoms Checklist: **Rate Symptoms 0-10**

- [ ] Headache
- [ ] Joint pain
- [ ] Muscle pain
- [ ] Other: _____
- [ ] Digestive symptoms
- [x] Abdominal pain
- [ ] Tinnitus
- [ ] Other: _____

Energy level: 4
Mood: 10
Mental Clarity: 8
Purpose/Hope: 10

13

Date _____ June 13, 2022 _____

❑ FCLO/HVBO	☒ Probiotic	❑ Detox Bath	❑ AM Juicing	☒ Fat
☒ Omega 3/6	❑ Beet Kvass	❑ Oil Pull	❑ PM Juicing	❑ Stock
❑ Iodine	❑ Milk Kefir	☒ Sunbathing	☒ Movement	☒ Ferments

Take a Moment:

There can be no vulnerability without risk; there can be no community without vulnerability; there can be no peace, and ultimately no life, without community. —M. Scott Peck

Are you part of a community where you can be vulnerable? If not, where could you find one?
I am not. I guess I need to take a look.

Today's Focus: Wash my body

Nutritional Intake:

Breakfast 2-eggs - blueberries - yogurt 2-Almond flour pancakes w/ Honey 2-organ supplements; coffee w/ collagen

Mid-morning _____

Lunch Deer stew w/ spinach, w/ Duck fat & surkraut. 2 organ supplements

Mid-afternoon _____

Dinner 2 organ supplements

Evening _____

New Foods/Reactions: _____

Stools (amount, number and type): not full movement, #3

Quick Symptoms Checklist: Rate Symptoms 0-10

❑ Headache	❑ Digestive symptoms	Energy level: 7
❑ Joint pain	❑ Abdominal pain	Mood: 10
❑ Muscle pain	❑ Tinnitus	Mental Clarity: 7
❑ Other: _____	❑ Other: _____	Purpose/Hope: 10

14

166 lbs.

Date June 14, 2022

- ☐ FCLO/HVBO
- ☑ Omega 3/6
- ☐ Iodine
- ☐ Probiotic
- ☐ Beet Kvass
- ☐ Milk Kefir
- ☐ Detox Bath
- ☐ Oil Pull
- ☑ Sunbathing
- ☐ AM Juicing
- ☐ PM Juicing
- ☑ Movement
- ☑ Fat
- ☑ Stock
- ☑ Ferments

Take a Moment:

A goal without a plan is just a wish. —Antoine de Saint-Exupéry

Think of a goal. What is your plan to get it?

My goal is to achieve optimal health.
My plan is to keep nurishing my body
with organic whole food, move my
body and focus on rest/stress management.

Today's Focus: work at after work while sun
bathing

Nutritional Intake:

Breakfast 2-eggs - Blueberries - yogurt
2- Almond flur pancakes w/ Honey
2-argan supplements; coffee w/ collagen

Mid-morning ___

Lunch Deer stew w/ spinach w/ duck fart & 2 argan
supplements

Mid-afternoon ___

Dinner 2-argan supplements

Evening ___

New Foods/Reactions: Bloating today. 2-days before
period;

Stools (amount, number and type): #6

Quick Symptoms Checklist: **Rate Symptoms 0-10**

- ☐ Headache
- ☐ Joint pain
- ☐ Muscle pain
- ☐ Other: ___
- ☑ Digestive symptoms Heartburn tight pores.
- ☐ Abdominal pain
- ☐ Tinnitus
- ☐ Other: ___
- Energy level: 7
- Mood: 9
- Mental Clarity: 9
- Purpose/Hope: 10

15

Date June 15, 2022

- ❏ FCLO/HVBO
- ❏ Omega 3/6
- ❏ Iodine
- ❏ Probiotic
- ❏ Beet Kvass
- ❏ Milk Kefir
- ❏ Detox Bath
- ❏ Oil Pull
- ❏ Sunbathing
- ❏ AM Juicing
- ❏ PM Juicing
- ❏ Movement
- ❏ Fat
- ❏ Stock
- ❏ Ferments

Take a Moment:

Nobody made a greater mistake than he who did nothing because he could do only a little. —Edmund Burke

Do you feel like your progress will be too slow?
What value will come from the little steps you can make?

I think my progress is on point. I am taking it day by day, one step at a time.

Today's Focus: Hydration & Fat!

Nutritional Intake:

Breakfast _Same as prev. day_

Mid-morning _____

Lunch _Same as prev day_

Mid-afternoon _____

Dinner _Tequila tasting (sip) App. Tasting_

Evening _____

New Foods/Reactions: _____

Stools (amount, number and type): _____

Quick Symptoms Checklist: Rate Symptoms 0-10

- ❏ Headache
- ❏ Joint pain
- ❏ Muscle pain
- ❏ Other: _____
- ❏ Digestive symptoms
- ❏ Abdominal pain
- ❏ Tinnitus
- ❏ Other: _____

Energy level: _____
Mood: _____
Mental Clarity: _____
Purpose/Hope: _____

My week overall: 0--+--------------10

I would describe my week (in one word) as: Progress

Because? Made me #1; focused on Adria's nutrition and sleep.

General progress:

Advanced to a new stage? Y/N   Current stage? Full Gaps

New foods tolerated: All Added   Foods removed: ——

Animal fats consumed: Duck Lard   Avg. daily amount: 4 tbsp

# of days stock consumed: 7   Avg. daily amount: 1 cup
Soup

Probiotics/fermented foods/cultured dairy:

Probiotic supplement: ——————   Current dose: ——

Die-off symptoms Y/N   Describe: On Saturday 6/11 night.
diarreah.

Beet Kvass ——————   Sour Cream ——————

Veggie Medley ——————   Yogurt Yes

Sauerkraut Yes   Kefir ——————

Detoxing Progress:

# of detox baths: 1   Ingredients: ACV/Epsom/Baking soda

# of days sunbathed: 2   # of minutes per session: 30 minutes

# of days juiced in am: ——————   in pm: ——————

Ingredients: _____

Overall reactions to detoxing: None

Symptoms descriptions:

Stools: Daily Y/N   #per day 1   Type(s): mostly loose

Digestion: Much better; longer between meals

Mood/energy: Great; stable blood sugar.

Memory/clarity: Some

Sleep/Stress: Less stress more sleep.

Typical-for-me symptoms: Fatigue but its improving

Date 6/16

❏ FCLO/HVBO	❏ Probiotic	❏ Detox Bath	❏ AM Juicing	❏ Fat
❏ Omega 3/6	❏ Beet Kvass	❏ Oil Pull	❏ PM Juicing	❏ Stock
❏ Iodine	❏ Milk Kefir	❏ Sunbathing	❏ Movement	❏ Ferments

Take a Moment:

Far away there in the sunshine are my highest aspirations. I may not reach them, but I can look up and see their beauty, believe in them, and try to follow them. —Louisa May Alcott

What high aspiration do you believe in, or want to believe in, for yourself?

That I can achieve optimal health for me.

Today's Focus: Nutrition

Nutritional Intake:

Breakfast _Same as prev day_

Mid-morning _____

Lunch _Same as prev day w/_ Zucchini

Mid-afternoon _____

Dinner _____

Evening _____

New Foods/Reactions: _____

Stools (amount, number and type): _____

Quick Symptoms Checklist: Rate Symptoms 0-10

❏ Headache	❏ Digestive symptoms	Energy level:_____
❏ Joint pain	❏ Abdominal pain	Mood: _____
❏ Muscle pain	❏ Tinnitus	Mental Clarity: _____
❏ Other: _____	❏ Other: _____	Purpose/Hope: _____

Date ___6 | 17___

- ☐ FCLO/HVBO
- ☐ Omega 3/6
- ☐ Iodine
- ☐ Probiotic
- ☐ Beet Kvass
- ☐ Milk Kefir
- ☐ Detox Bath
- ☐ Oil Pull
- ☐ Sunbathing
- ☑ AM Juicing
- ☑ PM Juicing
- ☐ Movement
- ☑ Fat
- ☐ Stock
- ☑ Ferments

Take a Moment:

All you have to do is look straight and see the road,
and when you see it, don't sit looking at it--walk. —Ayn Rand

How can you walk forward today?

Stay on the path. Left work early, sick
maybe COVID. Stay w/ diet 100%

Today's Focus: Nutrition

Nutritional Intake:

Breakfast _Same as prev day_

Mid-morning _____

Lunch _Sunflower butter; banana; Honey; sea salt._

Mid-afternoon _2 eggs; Elderberry tea._

Dinner _Salmon; zucchini; string beans._

Evening _____

New Foods/Reactions: _____

Stools (amount, number and type): _# 6_

Quick Symptoms Checklist: **Rate Symptoms 0-10**

☑ Headache	☐ Digestive symptoms	Energy level: 4
☑ Joint pain	☐ Abdominal pain	Mood: 6
☑ Muscle pain	☐ Tinnitus	Mental Clarity: 6
☑ Other: sinus	☐ Other: _____	Purpose/Hope: 10

Date __6/18/2022__

❏ FCLO/HVBO	❏ Probiotic	❏ Detox Bath	❏ AM Juicing	❏ Fat
❏ Omega 3/6	❏ Beet Kvass	❏ Oil Pull	❏ PM Juicing	❏ Stock
❏ Iodine	❏ Milk Kefir	❏ Sunbathing	❏ Movement	❏ Ferments

Take a Moment:

One resolution I have made, and try always to keep, is this: To rise above the little things. —John Burroughs

What little things are hindering your sucess?
How can you rise above them?

Motivation to workout or go for a walk. Set up the house for success.

Today's Focus: _Cleaning the house & meal prep for tomorrow._

Nutritional Intake:

Breakfast _____

Mid-morning _____

Lunch _____

Mid-afternoon _____

Dinner _____

Evening _____

New Foods/Reactions: _____

Stools (amount, number and type): _____

Quick Symptoms Checklist: Rate Symptoms 0-10

❏ Headache	❏ Digestive symptoms	Energy level:_____
❏ Joint pain	❏ Abdominal pain	Mood: _____
❏ Muscle pain	❏ Tinnitus	Mental Clarity: _____
❏ Other: _____	❏ Other: _____	Purpose/Hope: _____

Date _____

❏ FCLO/HVBO	❏ Probiotic	❏ Detox Bath	❏ AM Juicing	❏ Fat
❏ Omega 3/6	❏ Beet Kvass	❏ Oil Pull	❏ PM Juicing	❏ Stock
❏ Iodine	❏ Milk Kefir	❏ Sunbathing	❏ Movement	❏ Ferments

Take a Moment:

If a man will begin with certainties, he shall end in doubts, but if he will be content to begin with doubts, he shall end in certainties.
—Sir Francis Bacon

Do you have doubts about what you are doing?

_____

_____

Today's Focus: _____

Nutritional Intake:

Breakfast _____

Mid-morning_____

Lunch _____

Mid-afternoon _____

Dinner _____

Evening _____

New Foods/Reactions: _____

Stools (amount, number and type): _____

_____

Quick Symptoms Checklist: **Rate Symptoms 0-10**

❏ Headache	❏ Digestive symptoms	Energy level:_____
❏ Joint pain	❏ Abdominal pain	Mood: _____
❏ Muscle pain	❏ Tinnitus	Mental Clarity: _____
❏ Other: _____	❏ Other: _____	Purpose/Hope: _____

Date _____

❏ FCLO/HVBO	❏ Probiotic	❏ Detox Bath	❏ AM Juicing	❏ Fat
❏ Omega 3/6	❏ Beet Kvass	❏ Oil Pull	❏ PM Juicing	❏ Stock
❏ Iodine	❏ Milk Kefir	❏ Sunbathing	❏ Movement	❏ Ferments

Take a Moment:

You have to leave the city of your comfort and go into the wilderness of your intuition. What you'll discover will be wonderful. What you'll discover is yourself. —Alan Alda

Part of this health journey is learning to listen to your intuition. What have you learned?

_____

_____

Today's Focus: _____

Nutritional Intake:

Breakfast _____

Mid-morning_____

Lunch _____

Mid-afternoon _____

Dinner _____

Evening _____

New Foods/Reactions: _____

Stools (amount, number and type): _____

_____

Quick Symptoms Checklist:		**Rate Symptoms 0-10**
❏ Headache	❏ Digestive symptoms	Energy level:_____
❏ Joint pain	❏ Abdominal pain	Mood: _____
❏ Muscle pain	❏ Tinnitus	Mental Clarity: _____
❏ Other: _____	❏ Other: _____	Purpose/Hope: _____

Date _____

❏ FCLO/HVBO	❏ Probiotic	❏ Detox Bath	❏ AM Juicing	❏ Fat
❏ Omega 3/6	❏ Beet Kvass	❏ Oil Pull	❏ PM Juicing	❏ Stock
❏ Iodine	❏ Milk Kefir	❏ Sunbathing	❏ Movement	❏ Ferments

Take a Moment:

Ideals are like the stars; we never reach them, but like the mariners of the sea, we chart our course by them. —Carl Schurz

How do you balance ideals versus realities?

_____

_____

_____

Today's Focus: _____

Nutritional Intake:

Breakfast _____

Mid-morning_____

Lunch _____

Mid-afternoon _____

Dinner _____

Evening _____

New Foods/Reactions: _____

Stools (amount, number and type): _____

_____

Quick Symptoms Checklist: Rate Symptoms 0-10

❏ Headache	❏ Digestive symptoms	Energy level:_____
❏ Joint pain	❏ Abdominal pain	Mood: _____
❏ Muscle pain	❏ Tinnitus	Mental Clarity: _____
❏ Other: _____	❏ Other: _____	Purpose/Hope: _____

Date _____

❏ FCLO/HVBO	❏ Probiotic	❏ Detox Bath	❏ AM Juicing	❏ Fat
❏ Omega 3/6	❏ Beet Kvass	❏ Oil Pull	❏ PM Juicing	❏ Stock
❏ Iodine	❏ Milk Kefir	❏ Sunbathing	❏ Movement	❏ Ferments

Take a Moment:

Make voyages! Attempt them! There's nothing else.
—Tennessee Williams

Do you feel aftaid of the failing the journey?
Should you go on anyway?

_____
_____

Today's Focus: _____

Nutritional Intake:

Breakfast _____

Mid-morning_____

Lunch _____

Mid-afternoon _____

Dinner _____

Evening _____

New Foods/Reactions: _____

Stools (amount, number and type): _____

Quick Symptoms Checklist:		**Rate Symptoms 0-10**
❏ Headache	❏ Digestive symptoms	Energy level:_____
❏ Joint pain	❏ Abdominal pain	Mood: _____
❏ Muscle pain	❏ Tinnitus	Mental Clarity:_____
❏ Other: _____	❏ Other: _____	Purpose/Hope: _____

My week overall: 0---10

I would describe my week (in one word) as: _____

Because? _____

General progress:

Advanced to a new stage? Y/N Current stage?_____

New foods tolerated: _____ Foods removed: _____

Animal fats consumed: _____ Avg. daily amount: _____

# of days stock consumed: _____ Avg. daily amount: _____

Probiotics/fermented foods/cultured dairy:

Probiotic supplement: _____Current dose: _____

Die-off symptoms: Y/N Describe: _____

_____

Beet Kvass_____ Sour Cream_____

Veggie Medley_____ Yogurt _____

Sauerkraut_____ Kefir_____

Detoxing Progress:

# of detox baths: _____ Ingredients: ACV/Epsom/Baking soda

# of days sunbathed: _____ # of minutes per session:_____ minutes

# of days juiced in am: _____in pm: _____

Ingredients:_____

Overall reactions to detoxing: _____

Symptoms descriptions:

Stools: Daily Y/N   #per day _____   Type(s):_____

Digestion: _____

Mood/energy: _____

Memory/clarity: _____

Sleep/Stress: _____

Typical-for-me symptoms: _____

_____

Date _____

❑ FCLO/HVBO	❑ Probiotic	❑ Detox Bath	❑ AM Juicing	❑ Fat
❑ Omega 3/6	❑ Beet Kvass	❑ Oil Pull	❑ PM Juicing	❑ Stock
❑ Iodine	❑ Milk Kefir	❑ Sunbathing	❑ Movement	❑ Ferments

Take a Moment:

The real sin against life is to abuse and destory beauty, even one's own—even more, one's own, for that has been put in our care and we are responsible for its well-being. —Katherine Anne Porter

Is there something you are doing that is destroying your own beauty? Can you resolve to stop doing it today?

_____

_____

Today's Focus: _____

Nutritional Intake:

Breakfast _____

Mid-morning_____

Lunch _____

Mid-afternoon _____

Dinner _____

Evening _____

New Foods/Reactions:_____

Stools (amount, number and type): _____

_____

Quick Symptoms Checklist: **Rate Symptoms 0-10**

❑ Headache	❑ Digestive symptoms	Energy level:_____
❑ Joint pain	❑ Abdominal pain	Mood: _____
❑ Muscle pain	❑ Tinnitus	Mental Clarity: _____
❑ Other: _____	❑ Other: _____	Purpose/Hope: _____

Date _____

❏ FCLO/HVBO	❏ Probiotic	❏ Detox Bath	❏ AM Juicing	❏ Fat
❏ Omega 3/6	❏ Beet Kvass	❏ Oil Pull	❏ PM Juicing	❏ Stock
❏ Iodine	❏ Milk Kefir	❏ Sunbathing	❏ Movement	❏ Ferments

Take a Moment:

You cannot make yourself feel something you do not feel, but you can make yourself do right in spite of your feelings. —Pearl S. Buck

What is something you can do right today, despite how you feel?

_____

_____

_____

Today's Focus: _____

Nutritional Intake:

Breakfast _____

Mid-morning_____

Lunch _____

Mid-afternoon _____

Dinner _____

Evening _____

New Foods/Reactions: _____

Stools (amount, number and type): _____

_____

Quick Symptoms Checklist: **Rate Symptoms 0-10**

❏ Headache	❏ Digestive symptoms	Energy level:_____
❏ Joint pain	❏ Abdominal pain	Mood: _____
❏ Muscle pain	❏ Tinnitus	Mental Clarity:_____
❏ Other: _____	❏ Other: _____	Purpose/Hope: _____

Date _____

❑ FCLO/HVBO	❑ Probiotic	❑ Detox Bath	❑ AM Juicing	❑ Fat
❑ Omega 3/6	❑ Beet Kvass	❑ Oil Pull	❑ PM Juicing	❑ Stock
❑ Iodine	❑ Milk Kefir	❑ Sunbathing	❑ Movement	❑ Ferments

Take a Moment:

Success is the ability to go from one failure to another with no loss of enthusiasm. —Sir Winston Churchill

How do you keep your enthusiasm?

_____

_____

_____

Today's Focus: _____

Nutritional Intake:

Breakfast _____

Mid-morning_____

Lunch _____

Mid-afternoon _____

Dinner _____

Evening _____

New Foods/Reactions: _____

Stools (amount, number and type): _____

Quick Symptoms Checklist:		Rate Symptoms 0-10
❑ Headache	❑ Digestive symptoms	Energy level:_____
❑ Joint pain	❑ Abdominal pain	Mood: _____
❑ Muscle pain	❑ Tinnitus	Mental Clarity: _____
❑ Other: _____	❑ Other: _____	Purpose/Hope: _____

Date _____

❏ FCLO/HVBO	❏ Probiotic	❏ Detox Bath	❏ AM Juicing	❏ Fat
❏ Omega 3/6	❏ Beet Kvass	❏ Oil Pull	❏ PM Juicing	❏ Stock
❏ Iodine	❏ Milk Kefir	❏ Sunbathing	❏ Movement	❏ Ferments

Take a Moment:

If you really want to do something, you'll find a way.
If you don't, you'll find an excuse. —Jim Rohn

Are you finding ways or excuses?

_____

_____

_____

Today's Focus: _____

Nutritional Intake:

Breakfast _____

Mid-morning_____

Lunch _____

Mid-afternoon _____

Dinner _____

Evening _____

New Foods/Reactions: _____

Stools (amount, number and type): _____

_____

Quick Symptoms Checklist:		**Rate Symptoms 0-10**
❏ Headache	❏ Digestive symptoms	Energy level:_____
❏ Joint pain	❏ Abdominal pain	Mood: _____
❏ Muscle pain	❏ Tinnitus	Mental Clarity:_____
❏ Other: _____	❏ Other: _____	Purpose/Hope: _____

Date _____

❏ FCLO/HVBO	❏ Probiotic	❏ Detox Bath	❏ AM Juicing	❏ Fat
❏ Omega 3/6	❏ Beet Kvass	❏ Oil Pull	❏ PM Juicing	❏ Stock
❏ Iodine	❏ Milk Kefir	❏ Sunbathing	❏ Movement	❏ Ferments

Take a Moment:

He who has a why to live for can bear almost any how.
—Friedrich Nietzsche

What is your why?

_____

_____

_____

Today's Focus: _____

Nutritional Intake:

Breakfast _____

Mid-morning _____

Lunch _____

Mid-afternoon _____

Dinner _____

Evening _____

New Foods/Reactions: _____

Stools (amount, number and type): _____

Quick Symptoms Checklist: **Rate Symptoms 0-10**

❏ Headache	❏ Digestive symptoms	Energy level:_____
❏ Joint pain	❏ Abdominal pain	Mood: _____
❏ Muscle pain	❏ Tinnitus	Mental Clarity: _____
❏ Other: _____	❏ Other: _____	Purpose/Hope: ____

Date _____

❏ FCLO/HVBO	❏ Probiotic	❏ Detox Bath	❏ AM Juicing	❏ Fat
❏ Omega 3/6	❏ Beet Kvass	❏ Oil Pull	❏ PM Juicing	❏ Stock
❏ Iodine	❏ Milk Kefir	❏ Sunbathing	❏ Movement	❏ Ferments

Take a Moment:

Hope costs nothing. —Colette

What do you think about this? Does it feel true in your life, or not?

_____

_____

_____

Today's Focus: _____

Nutritional Intake:

Breakfast _____

Mid-morning _____

Lunch _____

Mid-afternoon _____

Dinner _____

Evening _____

New Foods/Reactions: _____

Stools (amount, number and type): _____

_____

Quick Symptoms Checklist:		**Rate Symptoms 0-10**
❏ Headache	❏ Digestive symptoms	Energy level:_____
❏ Joint pain	❏ Abdominal pain	Mood: _____
❏ Muscle pain	❏ Tinnitus	Mental Clarity: _____
❏ Other: _____	❏ Other: _____	Purpose/Hope: _____

Date _____

❑ FCLO/HVBO	❑ Probiotic	❑ Detox Bath	❑ AM Juicing	❑ Fat
❑ Omega 3/6	❑ Beet Kvass	❑ Oil Pull	❑ PM Juicing	❑ Stock
❑ Iodine	❑ Milk Kefir	❑ Sunbathing	❑ Movement	❑ Ferments

Take a Moment:

Though no one can go back and make a brand new start, anyone can start from now and make a brand new ending. —Carl Bard

What new ending do you want to start making from now?

_____

_____

_____

Today's Focus: _____

Nutritional Intake:

Breakfast _____

Mid-morning_____

Lunch _____

Mid-afternoon _____

Dinner _____

Evening _____

New Foods/Reactions: _____

Stools (amount, number and type): _____

Quick Symptoms Checklist: **Rate Symptoms 0-10**

❑ Headache	❑ Digestive symptoms	Energy level:_____
❑ Joint pain	❑ Abdominal pain	Mood: _____
❑ Muscle pain	❑ Tinnitus	Mental Clarity: _____
❑ Other: _____	❑ Other: _____	Purpose/Hope: ____

Date _____

My week overall: 0--10

I would describe my week (in one word) as: _____

Because? _____

General progress:

Advanced to a new stage? Y/N   Current stage?_____

New foods tolerated: _____   Foods removed: _____

Animal fats consumed: _____   Avg. daily amount: _____

# of days stock consumed: _____   Avg. daily amount: _____

Probiotics/fermented foods/cultured dairy:

Probiotic supplement: _____Current dose: _____

Die-off symptoms: Y/N   Describe: _____

_____

Beet Kvass _____   Sour Cream _____

Veggie Medley_____   Yogurt _____

Sauerkraut_____   Kefir_____

Detoxing Progress:

# of detox baths: _____ Ingredients: ACV/Epsom/Baking soda

# of days sunbathed: _____ # of minutes per session:_____ minutes

# of days juiced in am: _____in pm: _____

Ingredients:_____

Overall reactions to detoxing: _____

Symptoms descriptions:

Stools: Daily Y/N   #per day _____   Type(s):_____

Digestion: _____

Mood/energy: _____

Memory/clarity: _____

Sleep/Stress: _____

Typical-for-me symptoms: _____

_____

Date _____

❑ FCLO/HVBO	❑ Probiotic	❑ Detox Bath	❑ AM Juicing	❑ Fat
❑ Omega 3/6	❑ Beet Kvass	❑ Oil Pull	❑ PM Juicing	❑ Stock
❑ Iodine	❑ Milk Kefir	❑ Sunbathing	❑ Movement	❑ Ferments

Take a Moment:

It is our attitude at the beginning of a difficult task which, more than anything else, will affect its successful outcome. —William James

How is your attitude?

_____

_____

_____

Today's Focus: _____

Nutritional Intake:

Breakfast _____

Mid-morning _____

Lunch _____

Mid-afternoon _____

Dinner _____

Evening _____

New Foods/Reactions: _____

Stools (amount, number and type): _____

_____

Quick Symptoms Checklist: Rate Symptoms 0-10

❑ Headache	❑ Digestive symptoms	Energy level:_____
❑ Joint pain	❑ Abdominal pain	Mood: _____
❑ Muscle pain	❑ Tinnitus	Mental Clarity: _____
❑ Other: _____	❑ Other: _____	Purpose/Hope: _____

Date _____

❑ FCLO/HVBO	❑ Probiotic	❑ Detox Bath	❑ AM Juicing	❑ Fat
❑ Omega 3/6	❑ Beet Kvass	❑ Oil Pull	❑ PM Juicing	❑ Stock
❑ Iodine	❑ Milk Kefir	❑ Sunbathing	❑ Movement	❑ Ferments

Take a Moment:

Mistakes are part of the dues one pays for a full life. —Sophia Loren

Are you missing out on living because you are afraid of making a mistake?

_____

_____

_____

Today's Focus: _____

Nutritional Intake:

Breakfast _____

Mid-morning_____

Lunch _____

Mid-afternoon _____

Dinner _____

Evening _____

New Foods/Reactions:_____

Stools (amount, number and type): _____

_____

Quick Symptoms Checklist: **Rate Symptoms 0-10**

❑ Headache	❑ Digestive symptoms	Energy level:_____
❑ Joint pain	❑ Abdominal pain	Mood: _____
❑ Muscle pain	❑ Tinnitus	Mental Clarity: _____
❑ Other: _____	❑ Other: _____	Purpose/Hope: _____

Date _____

❑ FCLO/HVBO	❑ Probiotic	❑ Detox Bath	❑ AM Juicing	❑ Fat
❑ Omega 3/6	❑ Beet Kvass	❑ Oil Pull	❑ PM Juicing	❑ Stock
❑ Iodine	❑ Milk Kefir	❑ Sunbathing	❑ Movement	❑ Ferments

Take a Moment:

To make no mistake is not in the power of man; but from their errors and mistakes the wise and good learn wisdom for the future.
—Plutarch

What have you learned from a recent mistake?

_____

_____

_____

Today's Focus: _____

Nutritional Intake:

Breakfast _____

Mid-morning_____

Lunch _____

Mid-afternoon _____

Dinner _____

Evening _____

New Foods/Reactions: _____

Stools (amount, number and type): _____

_____

Quick Symptoms Checklist: Rate Symptoms 0-10

❑ Headache	❑ Digestive symptoms	Energy level:_____
❑ Joint pain	❑ Abdominal pain	Mood: _____
❑ Muscle pain	❑ Tinnitus	Mental Clarity: _____
❑ Other: _____	❑ Other: _____	Purpose/Hope: _____

Date _____

❑ FCLO/HVBO	❑ Probiotic	❑ Detox Bath	❑ AM Juicing	❑ Fat
❑ Omega 3/6	❑ Beet Kvass	❑ Oil Pull	❑ PM Juicing	❑ Stock
❑ Iodine	❑ Milk Kefir	❑ Sunbathing	❑ Movement	❑ Ferments

Take a Moment:

I can live for two months on a good compliment. —Mark Twain

Have you received a complement that supported you for a long time? Can you pass that on?

_____

_____

_____

Today's Focus: _____

Nutritional Intake:

Breakfast _____

Mid-morning_____

Lunch _____

Mid-afternoon _____

Dinner _____

Evening _____

New Foods/Reactions: _____

Stools (amount, number and type): _____

_____

Quick Symptoms Checklist:		**Rate Symptoms 0-10**
❑ Headache	❑ Digestive symptoms	Energy level:_____
❑ Joint pain	❑ Abdominal pain	Mood: _____
❑ Muscle pain	❑ Tinnitus	Mental Clarity: _____
❑ Other: _____	❑ Other: _____	Purpose/Hope: _____

Date _____

❏ FCLO/HVBO	❏ Probiotic	❏ Detox Bath	❏ AM Juicing	❏ Fat
❏ Omega 3/6	❏ Beet Kvass	❏ Oil Pull	❏ PM Juicing	❏ Stock
❏ Iodine	❏ Milk Kefir	❏ Sunbathing	❏ Movement	❏ Ferments

Take a Moment:

Not everything that is faced can be changed, but nothing can be changed until it is faced. —James Baldwin

What do you want to change that you are afraid to face?

_____

_____

_____

Today's Focus: _____

Nutritional Intake:

Breakfast _____

Mid-morning_____

Lunch _____

Mid-afternoon _____

Dinner _____

Evening _____

New Foods/Reactions:_____

Stools (amount, number and type): _____

_____

Quick Symptoms Checklist: **Rate Symptoms 0-10**

❏ Headache	❏ Digestive symptoms	Energy level:_____
❏ Joint pain	❏ Abdominal pain	Mood: _____
❏ Muscle pain	❏ Tinnitus	Mental Clarity:_____
❏ Other: _____	❏ Other: _____	Purpose/Hope: _____

Date _____

❏ FCLO/HVBO	❏ Probiotic	❏ Detox Bath	❏ AM Juicing	❏ Fat
❏ Omega 3/6	❏ Beet Kvass	❏ Oil Pull	❏ PM Juicing	❏ Stock
❏ Iodine	❏ Milk Kefir	❏ Sunbathing	❏ Movement	❏ Ferments

Take a Moment:

All growth is a leap in the dark, a spontaneous, unpremeditated act without benefit of experience. —Henry Miller

Do you feel like you have no idea what you are doing?
Think of a time that a leap in the dark resulted in growth.

_____
_____
_____

Today's Focus: _____

Nutritional Intake:

Breakfast _____

Mid-morning_____

Lunch _____

Mid-afternoon _____

Dinner _____

Evening _____

New Foods/Reactions: _____

Stools (amount, number and type): _____

_____

Quick Symptoms Checklist: **Rate Symptoms 0-10**

❏ Headache	❏ Digestive symptoms	Energy level:_____
❏ Joint pain	❏ Abdominal pain	Mood: _____
❏ Muscle pain	❏ Tinnitus	Mental Clarity:_____
❏ Other: _____	❏ Other: _____	Purpose/Hope: _____

Date _____

❏ FCLO/HVBO	❏ Probiotic	❏ Detox Bath	❏ AM Juicing	❏ Fat
❏ Omega 3/6	❏ Beet Kvass	❏ Oil Pull	❏ PM Juicing	❏ Stock
❏ Iodine	❏ Milk Kefir	❏ Sunbathing	❏ Movement	❏ Ferments

Take a Moment:

To be interested in the changing seasons is a happier state of mind than to be hopelessly in love with spring. —George Santayana

It can be scary and hard to change. What changes have you seen in yourself that are hard to accept?

_____

_____

Today's Focus: _____

Nutritional Intake:

Breakfast _____

Mid-morning_____

Lunch _____

Mid-afternoon _____

Dinner _____

Evening _____

New Foods/Reactions: _____

Stools (amount, number and type): _____

Quick Symptoms Checklist: | **Rate Symptoms 0-10**

❏ Headache	❏ Digestive symptoms	Energy level:_____
❏ Joint pain	❏ Abdominal pain	Mood: _____
❏ Muscle pain	❏ Tinnitus	Mental Clarity: _____
❏ Other: _____	❏ Other: _____	Purpose/Hope: _____

My week overall: 0--10

I would describe my week (in one word) as: _____

Because? _____

General progress:

Advanced to a new stage? Y/N   Current stage?_____

New foods tolerated: _____   Foods removed: _____

Animal fats consumed: _____   Avg. daily amount: _____

# of days stock consumed: _____   Avg. daily amount: _____

Probiotics/fermented foods/cultured dairy:

Probiotic supplement: _____Current dose: _____

Die-off symptoms: Y/N   Describe: _____

_____

Beet Kvass _____   Sour Cream _____

Veggie Medley_____   Yogurt _____

Sauerkraut_____   Kefir_____

Detoxing Progress:

# of detox baths: _____ Ingredients: ACV/Epsom/Baking soda

# of days sunbathed: _____ # of minutes per session:_____ minutes

# of days juiced in am: _____in pm: _____

Ingredients:_____

Overall reactions to detoxing: _____

Symptoms descriptions:

Stools: Daily Y/N   #per day _____   Type(s):_____

Digestion: _____

Mood/energy: _____

Memory/clarity: _____

Sleep/Stress: _____

Typical-for-me symptoms: _____

_____

Date _____

❑ FCLO/HVBO	❑ Probiotic	❑ Detox Bath	❑ AM Juicing	❑ Fat
❑ Omega 3/6	❑ Beet Kvass	❑ Oil Pull	❑ PM Juicing	❑ Stock
❑ Iodine	❑ Milk Kefir	❑ Sunbathing	❑ Movement	❑ Ferments

Take a Moment:

People, even more than things, have to be restored, renewed, revived, reclaimed, and redeemed; never throw out anyone. —Audrey Hepburn

You are worth reclaiming. Do you believe that you shouldn't be thrown out?

_____

_____

Today's Focus: _____

Nutritional Intake:

Breakfast _____

Mid-morning_____

Lunch _____

Mid-afternoon _____

Dinner _____

Evening _____

New Foods/Reactions: _____

Stools (amount, number and type): _____

Quick Symptoms Checklist: **Rate Symptoms 0-10**

❑ Headache	❑ Digestive symptoms	Energy level:_____
❑ Joint pain	❑ Abdominal pain	Mood: _____
❑ Muscle pain	❑ Tinnitus	Mental Clarity: _____
❑ Other: _____	❑ Other: _____	Purpose/Hope: _____

Date _____

❑ FCLO/HVBO	❑ Probiotic	❑ Detox Bath	❑ AM Juicing	❑ Fat
❑ Omega 3/6	❑ Beet Kvass	❑ Oil Pull	❑ PM Juicing	❑ Stock
❑ Iodine	❑ Milk Kefir	❑ Sunbathing	❑ Movement	❑ Ferments

Take a Moment:

The beginning is the most important part of the work. —Plato

How can you begin well?

_____

_____

_____

Today's Focus: _____

Nutritional Intake:

Breakfast _____

Mid-morning_____

Lunch _____

Mid-afternoon _____

Dinner _____

Evening _____

New Foods/Reactions: _____

Stools (amount, number and type): _____

Quick Symptoms Checklist: **Rate Symptoms 0-10**

❑ Headache	❑ Digestive symptoms	Energy level:_____
❑ Joint pain	❑ Abdominal pain	Mood: _____
❑ Muscle pain	❑ Tinnitus	Mental Clarity:_____
❑ Other: _____	❑ Other: _____	Purpose/Hope: _____

Date _____

❏ FCLO/HVBO	❏ Probiotic	❏ Detox Bath	❏ AM Juicing	❏ Fat
❏ Omega 3/6	❏ Beet Kvass	❏ Oil Pull	❏ PM Juicing	❏ Stock
❏ Iodine	❏ Milk Kefir	❏ Sunbathing	❏ Movement	❏ Ferments

Take a Moment:

If you want to go fast, go alone. If you want to go far, go together.
— African Proverb

Do you have support, so you can go far?

_____

_____

_____

Today's Focus: _____

Nutritional Intake:

Breakfast _____

Mid-morning _____

Lunch _____

Mid-afternoon _____

Dinner _____

Evening _____

New Foods/Reactions: _____

Stools (amount, number and type): _____

Quick Symptoms Checklist:		Rate Symptoms 0-10
❏ Headache	❏ Digestive symptoms	Energy level:_____
❏ Joint pain	❏ Abdominal pain	Mood: _____
❏ Muscle pain	❏ Tinnitus	Mental Clarity: _____
❏ Other: _____	❏ Other: _____	Purpose/Hope: _____

Date _____

❑ FCLO/HVBO	❑ Probiotic	❑ Detox Bath	❑ AM Juicing	❑ Fat
❑ Omega 3/6	❑ Beet Kvass	❑ Oil Pull	❑ PM Juicing	❑ Stock
❑ Iodine	❑ Milk Kefir	❑ Sunbathing	❑ Movement	❑ Ferments

Take a Moment:

Things do not change; we change. —Henry David Thoreau

Is there something you wished was different?
How can you change?

_____

_____

_____

Today's Focus: _____

Nutritional Intake:

Breakfast _____

Mid-morning_____

Lunch _____

Mid-afternoon _____

Dinner _____

Evening _____

New Foods/Reactions: _____

Stools (amount, number and type): _____

Quick Symptoms Checklist: **Rate Symptoms 0-10**

❑ Headache	❑ Digestive symptoms	Energy level:_____
❑ Joint pain	❑ Abdominal pain	Mood: _____
❑ Muscle pain	❑ Tinnitus	Mental Clarity: _____
❑ Other: _____	❑ Other: _____	Purpose/Hope: _____

Date _____

❏ FCLO/HVBO	❏ Probiotic	❏ Detox Bath	❏ AM Juicing	❏ Fat
❏ Omega 3/6	❏ Beet Kvass	❏ Oil Pull	❏ PM Juicing	❏ Stock
❏ Iodine	❏ Milk Kefir	❏ Sunbathing	❏ Movement	❏ Ferments

Take a Moment:

Nothing can stop the man with the right mental attitude from achieving his goal; nothing on earth can help the man with the wrong mental attitude. —Thomas Jefferson

What attitude do you have?

_____

_____

Today's Focus: _____

Nutritional Intake:

Breakfast _____

Mid-morning _____

Lunch _____

Mid-afternoon _____

Dinner _____

Evening _____

New Foods/Reactions: _____

Stools (amount, number and type): _____

_____

Quick Symptoms Checklist: Rate Symptoms 0-10

❏ Headache	❏ Digestive symptoms	Energy level:_____
❏ Joint pain	❏ Abdominal pain	Mood: _____
❏ Muscle pain	❏ Tinnitus	Mental Clarity: _____
❏ Other: _____	❏ Other: _____	Purpose/Hope: _____

Date _____

❏ FCLO/HVBO	❏ Probiotic	❏ Detox Bath	❏ AM Juicing	❏ Fat
❏ Omega 3/6	❏ Beet Kvass	❏ Oil Pull	❏ PM Juicing	❏ Stock
❏ Iodine	❏ Milk Kefir	❏ Sunbathing	❏ Movement	❏ Ferments

Take a Moment:

> *Nothing is particularly hard if you divide it into small jobs.*
> —Henry Ford

What seems too big to tackle? How can you divide it up?

_____

_____

_____

Today's Focus: _____

Nutritional Intake:

Breakfast _____

Mid-morning _____

Lunch _____

Mid-afternoon _____

Dinner _____

Evening _____

New Foods/Reactions: _____

Stools (amount, number and type): _____

_____

Quick Symptoms Checklist: **Rate Symptoms 0-10**

❏ Headache	❏ Digestive symptoms	Energy level:_____
❏ Joint pain	❏ Abdominal pain	Mood: _____
❏ Muscle pain	❏ Tinnitus	Mental Clarity: _____
❏ Other: _____	❏ Other: _____	Purpose/Hope: _____

Date _____

❑ FCLO/HVBO	❑ Probiotic	❑ Detox Bath	❑ AM Juicing	❑ Fat
❑ Omega 3/6	❑ Beet Kvass	❑ Oil Pull	❑ PM Juicing	❑ Stock
❑ Iodine	❑ Milk Kefir	❑ Sunbathing	❑ Movement	❑ Ferments

Take a Moment:

Tell me what you eat, and I will tell you what you are.
—Anthelme Brillat-Savarin

We are more than what we eat. What do you think he was talking about?

_____

_____

_____

Today's Focus: _____

Nutritional Intake:

Breakfast _____

Mid-morning _____

Lunch _____

Mid-afternoon _____

Dinner _____

Evening _____

New Foods/Reactions: _____

Stools (amount, number and type): _____

Quick Symptoms Checklist:		Rate Symptoms 0-10
❑ Headache	❑ Digestive symptoms	Energy level: _____
❑ Joint pain	❑ Abdominal pain	Mood: _____
❑ Muscle pain	❑ Tinnitus	Mental Clarity: _____
❑ Other: _____	❑ Other: _____	Purpose/Hope: _____

My week overall: 0--10

I would describe my week (in one word) as: _____

Because? _____

General progress:

Advanced to a new stage? Y/N   Current stage?_____

New foods tolerated: _____   Foods removed: _____

Animal fats consumed: _____   Avg. daily amount: _____

# of days stock consumed: _____   Avg. daily amount: _____

Probiotics/fermented foods/cultured dairy:

Probiotic supplement: _____Current dose: _____

Die-off symptoms: Y/N   Describe: _____

_____

Beet Kvass _____   Sour Cream _____

Veggie Medley_____   Yogurt _____

Sauerkraut_____   Kefir_____

Detoxing Progress:

# of detox baths: _____ Ingredients: ACV/Epsom/Baking soda

# of days sunbathed: _____ # of minutes per session:_____ minutes

# of days juiced in am: _____in pm: _____

Ingredients:_____

Overall reactions to detoxing: _____

Symptoms descriptions:

Stools: Daily Y/N   #per day _____   Type(s):_____

Digestion: _____

Mood/energy: _____

Memory/clarity: _____

Sleep/Stress: _____

Typical-for-me symptoms: _____

_____

Date _____

❏ FCLO/HVBO	❏ Probiotic	❏ Detox Bath	❏ AM Juicing	❏ Fat
❏ Omega 3/6	❏ Beet Kvass	❏ Oil Pull	❏ PM Juicing	❏ Stock
❏ Iodine	❏ Milk Kefir	❏ Sunbathing	❏ Movement	❏ Ferments

Take a Moment:

Every man takes the limits of his own field of vision for the limits of the world. —Arthur Schopenhauer

It's easy for us to think that what we see (or imagine) is all we can achieve. Write about something that seems beyond your limits.

_____

_____

_____

Today's Focus: _____

Nutritional Intake:

Breakfast _____

Mid-morning_____

Lunch _____

Mid-afternoon _____

Dinner _____

Evening _____

New Foods/Reactions: _____

Stools (amount, number and type): _____

_____

Quick Symptoms Checklist: **Rate Symptoms 0-10**

❏ Headache	❏ Digestive symptoms	Energy level:_____
❏ Joint pain	❏ Abdominal pain	Mood: _____
❏ Muscle pain	❏ Tinnitus	Mental Clarity: _____
❏ Other: _____	❏ Other: _____	Purpose/Hope: _____

Date _____

❑ FCLO/HVBO	❑ Probiotic	❑ Detox Bath	❑ AM Juicing	❑ Fat
❑ Omega 3/6	❑ Beet Kvass	❑ Oil Pull	❑ PM Juicing	❑ Stock
❑ Iodine	❑ Milk Kefir	❑ Sunbathing	❑ Movement	❑ Ferments

Take a Moment:

Change your thoughts and you change your world. —Norman Vincent Peale

What change of thought will you make today so that you can change your world?"

_____

_____

_____

Today's Focus: _____

Nutritional Intake:

Breakfast _____

Mid-morning _____

Lunch _____

Mid-afternoon _____

Dinner _____

Evening _____

New Foods/Reactions: _____

Stools (amount, number and type): _____

_____

Quick Symptoms Checklist: Rate Symptoms 0-10

❑ Headache	❑ Digestive symptoms	Energy level: _____
❑ Joint pain	❑ Abdominal pain	Mood: _____
❑ Muscle pain	❑ Tinnitus	Mental Clarity: _____
❑ Other: _____	❑ Other: _____	Purpose/Hope: _____

Date _____

❏ FCLO/HVBO	❏ Probiotic	❏ Detox Bath	❏ AM Juicing	❏ Fat
❏ Omega 3/6	❏ Beet Kvass	❏ Oil Pull	❏ PM Juicing	❏ Stock
❏ Iodine	❏ Milk Kefir	❏ Sunbathing	❏ Movement	❏ Ferments

Take a Moment:

Our life is frittered away by detail... simplify, simplify.
—Henry David Thoreau

What in your life can you simplify?

_____

_____

_____

Today's Focus: _____

Nutritional Intake:

Breakfast _____

Mid-morning _____

Lunch _____

Mid-afternoon _____

Dinner _____

Evening _____

New Foods/Reactions: _____

Stools (amount, number and type): _____

Quick Symptoms Checklist: **Rate Symptoms 0-10**

❏ Headache	❏ Digestive symptoms	Energy level: _____
❏ Joint pain	❏ Abdominal pain	Mood: _____
❏ Muscle pain	❏ Tinnitus	Mental Clarity: _____
❏ Other: _____	❏ Other: _____	Purpose/Hope: _____

Date _____

❏ FCLO/HVBO	❏ Probiotic	❏ Detox Bath	❏ AM Juicing	❏ Fat
❏ Omega 3/6	❏ Beet Kvass	❏ Oil Pull	❏ PM Juicing	❏ Stock
❏ Iodine	❏ Milk Kefir	❏ Sunbathing	❏ Movement	❏ Ferments

Take a Moment:

The self is not something ready-made, but something in continuous formation through choice of action. —John Dewey

What kind of self will your actions make today?

_____

_____

_____

Today's Focus: _____

Nutritional Intake:

Breakfast _____

Mid-morning_____

Lunch _____

Mid-afternoon _____

Dinner _____

Evening _____

New Foods/Reactions: _____

Stools (amount, number and type): _____

_____

Quick Symptoms Checklist: **Rate Symptoms 0-10**

❏ Headache	❏ Digestive symptoms	Energy level:_____
❏ Joint pain	❏ Abdominal pain	Mood: _____
❏ Muscle pain	❏ Tinnitus	Mental Clarity: _____
❏ Other: _____	❏ Other: _____	Purpose/Hope: _____

Date _____

❑ FCLO/HVBO	❑ Probiotic	❑ Detox Bath	❑ AM Juicing	❑ Fat
❑ Omega 3/6	❑ Beet Kvass	❑ Oil Pull	❑ PM Juicing	❑ Stock
❑ Iodine	❑ Milk Kefir	❑ Sunbathing	❑ Movement	❑ Ferments

Take a Moment:

When you blame others, you give up your power to change.
—Robert Anthony

Have you given up your power to change in an area?

_____

_____

_____

Today's Focus: _____

Nutritional Intake:

Breakfast _____

Mid-morning _____

Lunch _____

Mid-afternoon _____

Dinner _____

Evening _____

New Foods/Reactions: _____

Stools (amount, number and type): _____

Quick Symptoms Checklist: **Rate Symptoms 0-10**

❑ Headache	❑ Digestive symptoms	Energy level:_____
❑ Joint pain	❑ Abdominal pain	Mood: _____
❑ Muscle pain	❑ Tinnitus	Mental Clarity: _____
❑ Other: _____	❑ Other: _____	Purpose/Hope: _____

Date _____

❏ FCLO/HVBO	❏ Probiotic	❏ Detox Bath	❏ AM Juicing	❏ Fat
❏ Omega 3/6	❏ Beet Kvass	❏ Oil Pull	❏ PM Juicing	❏ Stock
❏ Iodine	❏ Milk Kefir	❏ Sunbathing	❏ Movement	❏ Ferments

Take a Moment:

You got to be careful if you don't know where you're going, because you might not get there. —Yogi Berra

Take a minute to remember where you are going.

_____

_____

_____

Today's Focus: _____

Nutritional Intake:

Breakfast _____

Mid-morning _____

Lunch _____

Mid-afternoon _____

Dinner _____

Evening _____

New Foods/Reactions: _____

Stools (amount, number and type): _____

_____

Quick Symptoms Checklist: Rate Symptoms 0-10

❏ Headache	❏ Digestive symptoms	Energy level: _____
❏ Joint pain	❏ Abdominal pain	Mood: _____
❏ Muscle pain	❏ Tinnitus	Mental Clarity: _____
❏ Other: _____	❏ Other: _____	Purpose/Hope: _____

Date _____

❏ FCLO/HVBO	❏ Probiotic	❏ Detox Bath	❏ AM Juicing	❏ Fat
❏ Omega 3/6	❏ Beet Kvass	❏ Oil Pull	❏ PM Juicing	❏ Stock
❏ Iodine	❏ Milk Kefir	❏ Sunbathing	❏ Movement	❏ Ferments

Take a Moment:

We have not passed that subtle line between childhood and adulthood until we move from the passive voice to the active voice--that is, until we have stopped saying, 'It got lost,' and say, 'I lost it.'
—Sydney J. Harris

How much responsibility do you take in your life?
_____
_____

Today's Focus: _____

Nutritional Intake:

Breakfast _____

Mid-morning_____

Lunch _____

Mid-afternoon _____

Dinner _____

Evening _____

New Foods/Reactions: _____

Stools (amount, number and type): _____

_____

Quick Symptoms Checklist:		Rate Symptoms 0-10
❏ Headache	❏ Digestive symptoms	Energy level:_____
❏ Joint pain	❏ Abdominal pain	Mood: _____
❏ Muscle pain	❏ Tinnitus	Mental Clarity: _____
❏ Other: _____	❏ Other: _____	Purpose/Hope: _____

My week overall: 0---10

I would describe my week (in one word) as: _____

Because? _____

General progress:

Advanced to a new stage? Y/N   Current stage?_____

New foods tolerated: _____   Foods removed: _____

Animal fats consumed: _____   Avg. daily amount: _____

# of days stock consumed: _____   Avg. daily amount: _____

Probiotics/fermented foods/cultured dairy:

Probiotic supplement: _____Current dose: _____

Die-off symptoms: Y/N   Describe: _____

_____

Beet Kvass _____   Sour Cream _____

Veggie Medley_____   Yogurt _____

Sauerkraut_____   Kefir_____

Detoxing Progress:

# of detox baths: _____ Ingredients: ACV/Epsom/Baking soda

# of days sunbathed: _____ # of minutes per session:_____ minutes

# of days juiced in am: _____in pm: _____

Ingredients:_____

Overall reactions to detoxing: _____

Symptoms descriptions:

Stools: Daily Y/N   #per day _____   Type(s):_____

Digestion: _____

Mood/energy: _____

Memory/clarity: _____

Sleep/Stress: _____

Typical-for-me symptoms: _____

_____

Date _____

❑ FCLO/HVBO	❑ Probiotic	❑ Detox Bath	❑ AM Juicing	❑ Fat
❑ Omega 3/6	❑ Beet Kvass	❑ Oil Pull	❑ PM Juicing	❑ Stock
❑ Iodine	❑ Milk Kefir	❑ Sunbathing	❑ Movement	❑ Ferments

Take a Moment:

Never be afraid to sit awhile and think. —Lorraine Hansbury

Write your plan to rest and be quiet sometime today.

_____

_____

_____

_____

Today's Focus: _____

Nutritional Intake:

Breakfast _____

Mid-morning_____

Lunch _____

Mid-afternoon _____

Dinner _____

Evening _____

New Foods/Reactions:_____

Stools (amount, number and type): _____

Quick Symptoms Checklist: **Rate Symptoms 0-10**

❑ Headache	❑ Digestive symptoms	Energy level:_____
❑ Joint pain	❑ Abdominal pain	Mood: _____
❑ Muscle pain	❑ Tinnitus	Mental Clarity: _____
❑ Other: _____	❑ Other: _____	Purpose/Hope: _____

Date _____

❑ FCLO/HVBO	❑ Probiotic	❑ Detox Bath	❑ AM Juicing	❑ Fat
❑ Omega 3/6	❑ Beet Kvass	❑ Oil Pull	❑ PM Juicing	❑ Stock
❑ Iodine	❑ Milk Kefir	❑ Sunbathing	❑ Movement	❑ Ferments

Take a Moment:

One kind word can warm three winter months. —Japanese Proverb

Who do you know that needs a kind word?
What will you say to them today?

_____

_____

_____

Today's Focus: _____

Nutritional Intake:

Breakfast _____

Mid-morning_____

Lunch _____

Mid-afternoon _____

Dinner _____

Evening _____

New Foods/Reactions: _____

Stools (amount, number and type): _____

_____

Quick Symptoms Checklist:		**Rate Symptoms 0-10**
❑ Headache	❑ Digestive symptoms	Energy level:_____
❑ Joint pain	❑ Abdominal pain	Mood: _____
❑ Muscle pain	❑ Tinnitus	Mental Clarity: _____
❑ Other: _____	❑ Other: _____	Purpose/Hope: _____

Date _____

❏ FCLO/HVBO	❏ Probiotic	❏ Detox Bath	❏ AM Juicing	❏ Fat
❏ Omega 3/6	❏ Beet Kvass	❏ Oil Pull	❏ PM Juicing	❏ Stock
❏ Iodine	❏ Milk Kefir	❏ Sunbathing	❏ Movement	❏ Ferments

Take a Moment:

*A river cuts through rock, not because of its power,
but because of its persistence.* —Jim Watkins

Persistence can be hard. How will you keep going?

_____

_____

_____

Today's Focus: _____

Nutritional Intake:

Breakfast _____

Mid-morning_____

Lunch _____

Mid-afternoon _____

Dinner _____

Evening _____

New Foods/Reactions:_____

Stools (amount, number and type): _____

Quick Symptoms Checklist: **Rate Symptoms 0-10**

❏ Headache	❏ Digestive symptoms	Energy level:_____
❏ Joint pain	❏ Abdominal pain	Mood: _____
❏ Muscle pain	❏ Tinnitus	Mental Clarity: _____
❏ Other: _____	❏ Other: _____	Purpose/Hope: _____

Date _____

❏ FCLO/HVBO	❏ Probiotic	❏ Detox Bath	❏ AM Juicing	❏ Fat
❏ Omega 3/6	❏ Beet Kvass	❏ Oil Pull	❏ PM Juicing	❏ Stock
❏ Iodine	❏ Milk Kefir	❏ Sunbathing	❏ Movement	❏ Ferments

Take a Moment:

I do not read advertisements. I would spend all of my time wanting things. —Franz Kafka

What are you keeping around that leaves you wanting?

_____

_____

_____

Today's Focus: _____

Nutritional Intake:

Breakfast _____

Mid-morning _____

Lunch _____

Mid-afternoon _____

Dinner _____

Evening _____

New Foods/Reactions: _____

Stools (amount, number and type): _____

_____

Quick Symptoms Checklist: **Rate Symptoms 0-10**

❏ Headache	❏ Digestive symptoms	Energy level:_____
❏ Joint pain	❏ Abdominal pain	Mood: _____
❏ Muscle pain	❏ Tinnitus	Mental Clarity:_____
❏ Other: _____	❏ Other: _____	Purpose/Hope: _____

Date _____

❏ FCLO/HVBO	❏ Probiotic	❏ Detox Bath	❏ AM Juicing	❏ Fat
❏ Omega 3/6	❏ Beet Kvass	❏ Oil Pull	❏ PM Juicing	❏ Stock
❏ Iodine	❏ Milk Kefir	❏ Sunbathing	❏ Movement	❏ Ferments

Take a Moment:

Better keep yourself clean and bright; you are the window through which you must see the world. —George Bernard Shaw

Depression and exhaustion are wearying. Have you experienced how getting up and moving will benefit you?

_____

_____

_____

Today's Focus: _____

Nutritional Intake:

Breakfast _____

Mid-morning_____

Lunch _____

Mid-afternoon _____

Dinner _____

Evening _____

New Foods/Reactions:_____

Stools (amount, number and type): _____

_____

Quick Symptoms Checklist:		**Rate Symptoms 0-10**
❏ Headache	❏ Digestive symptoms	Energy level:_____
❏ Joint pain	❏ Abdominal pain	Mood: _____
❏ Muscle pain	❏ Tinnitus	Mental Clarity: _____
❏ Other: _____	❏ Other: _____	Purpose/Hope: _____

Date _____

❑ FCLO/HVBO	❑ Probiotic	❑ Detox Bath	❑ AM Juicing	❑ Fat
❑ Omega 3/6	❑ Beet Kvass	❑ Oil Pull	❑ PM Juicing	❑ Stock
❑ Iodine	❑ Milk Kefir	❑ Sunbathing	❑ Movement	❑ Ferments

Take a Moment:

The unfortunate thing about this world is that the good habits are much easier to give up than the bad ones. —W. Somerset Maugham

What good habits have you given up doing?

_____

_____

_____

Today's Focus: _____

Nutritional Intake:

Breakfast _____

Mid-morning_____

Lunch _____

Mid-afternoon _____

Dinner _____

Evening _____

New Foods/Reactions: _____

Stools (amount, number and type): _____

_____

Quick Symptoms Checklist: Rate Symptoms 0-10

❑ Headache	❑ Digestive symptoms	Energy level:_____
❑ Joint pain	❑ Abdominal pain	Mood: _____
❑ Muscle pain	❑ Tinnitus	Mental Clarity:_____
❑ Other: _____	❑ Other: _____	Purpose/Hope: _____

Date _____

❏ FCLO/HVBO	❏ Probiotic	❏ Detox Bath	❏ AM Juicing	❏ Fat
❏ Omega 3/6	❏ Beet Kvass	❏ Oil Pull	❏ PM Juicing	❏ Stock
❏ Iodine	❏ Milk Kefir	❏ Sunbathing	❏ Movement	❏ Ferments

Take a Moment:

Nature does not hurry, yet everything is accomplished. —Lao Tzu

How much do you hurry? Take time to slow down today.

_____

_____

_____

_____

Today's Focus: _____

Nutritional Intake:

Breakfast _____

Mid-morning _____

Lunch _____

Mid-afternoon _____

Dinner _____

Evening _____

New Foods/Reactions: _____

Stools (amount, number and type): _____

Quick Symptoms Checklist: **Rate Symptoms 0-10**

❏ Headache	❏ Digestive symptoms	Energy level: _____
❏ Joint pain	❏ Abdominal pain	Mood: _____
❏ Muscle pain	❏ Tinnitus	Mental Clarity: _____
❏ Other: _____	❏ Other: _____	Purpose/Hope: _____

My week overall: 0---10

I would describe my week (in one word) as: _____

Because? _____

General progress:

Advanced to a new stage? Y/N   Current stage?_____

New foods tolerated: _____   Foods removed: _____

Animal fats consumed: _____   Avg. daily amount: _____

# of days stock consumed: _____   Avg. daily amount: _____

Probiotics/fermented foods/cultured dairy:

Probiotic supplement: _____Current dose: _____

Die-off symptoms: Y/N   Describe: _____

_____

Beet Kvass _____   Sour Cream _____

Veggie Medley_____   Yogurt _____

Sauerkraut_____   Kefir_____

Detoxing Progress:

# of detox baths: _____ Ingredients: ACV/Epsom/Baking soda

# of days sunbathed: _____ # of minutes per session:_____ minutes

# of days juiced in am: _____in pm: _____

Ingredients:_____

Overall reactions to detoxing: _____

Symptoms descriptions:

Stools: Daily Y/N   #per day _____   Type(s):_____

Digestion: _____

Mood/energy: _____

Memory/clarity: _____

Sleep/Stress: _____

Typical-for-me symptoms: _____

_____

Date _____

❑ FCLO/HVBO	❑ Probiotic	❑ Detox Bath	❑ AM Juicing	❑ Fat
❑ Omega 3/6	❑ Beet Kvass	❑ Oil Pull	❑ PM Juicing	❑ Stock
❑ Iodine	❑ Milk Kefir	❑ Sunbathing	❑ Movement	❑ Ferments

Take a Moment:

The really happy person is the one who can enjoy the scenery on a detour. —Anonymous

Do you feel like you are on a detour?
What is nice about the scenery where you are?

_____

_____

_____

Today's Focus: _____

Nutritional Intake:

Breakfast _____

Mid-morning _____

Lunch _____

Mid-afternoon _____

Dinner _____

Evening _____

New Foods/Reactions: _____

Stools (amount, number and type): _____

Quick Symptoms Checklist: **Rate Symptoms 0-10**

❑ Headache	❑ Digestive symptoms	Energy level:_____
❑ Joint pain	❑ Abdominal pain	Mood: _____
❑ Muscle pain	❑ Tinnitus	Mental Clarity:_____
❑ Other: _____	❑ Other: _____	Purpose/Hope: _____

Date _____

❑ FCLO/HVBO	❑ Probiotic	❑ Detox Bath	❑ AM Juicing	❑ Fat
❑ Omega 3/6	❑ Beet Kvass	❑ Oil Pull	❑ PM Juicing	❑ Stock
❑ Iodine	❑ Milk Kefir	❑ Sunbathing	❑ Movement	❑ Ferments

Take a Moment:

Laughter is the sun that drives winter from the human face.
—Victor Hugo

Tired of winter? Think about something that makes you laugh!

_____

_____

_____

Today's Focus: _____

Nutritional Intake:

Breakfast _____

Mid-morning _____

Lunch _____

Mid-afternoon _____

Dinner _____

Evening _____

New Foods/Reactions: _____

Stools (amount, number and type): _____

Quick Symptoms Checklist: **Rate Symptoms 0-10**

❑ Headache	❑ Digestive symptoms	Energy level: _____
❑ Joint pain	❑ Abdominal pain	Mood: _____
❑ Muscle pain	❑ Tinnitus	Mental Clarity: _____
❑ Other: _____	❑ Other: _____	Purpose/Hope: _____

Date _____

❏ FCLO/HVBO	❏ Probiotic	❏ Detox Bath	❏ AM Juicing	❏ Fat
❏ Omega 3/6	❏ Beet Kvass	❏ Oil Pull	❏ PM Juicing	❏ Stock
❏ Iodine	❏ Milk Kefir	❏ Sunbathing	❏ Movement	❏ Ferments

Take a Moment:

> *Every noble work is at first impossible.* —Thomas Carlyle

Are you now doing something you used to think impossible?
_____
_____
_____
_____

Today's Focus: _____

Nutritional Intake:

Breakfast _____

Mid-morning_____

Lunch _____

Mid-afternoon _____

Dinner _____

Evening _____

New Foods/Reactions: _____

Stools (amount, number and type): _____

Quick Symptoms Checklist: **Rate Symptoms 0-10**

❏ Headache	❏ Digestive symptoms	Energy level:_____
❏ Joint pain	❏ Abdominal pain	Mood: _____
❏ Muscle pain	❏ Tinnitus	Mental Clarity: _____
❏ Other: _____	❏ Other: _____	Purpose/Hope: _____

Date _____

❑ FCLO/HVBO	❑ Probiotic	❑ Detox Bath	❑ AM Juicing	❑ Fat
❑ Omega 3/6	❑ Beet Kvass	❑ Oil Pull	❑ PM Juicing	❑ Stock
❑ Iodine	❑ Milk Kefir	❑ Sunbathing	❑ Movement	❑ Ferments

Take a Moment:

It's faith in something and enthusiasm for something that makes life worth living. —Oliver Wendell Holmes

It's easy to lose faith and enthusiasm in life. Have you lost yours?

_____

_____

_____

Today's Focus: _____

Nutritional Intake:

Breakfast _____

Mid-morning_____

Lunch _____

Mid-afternoon _____

Dinner _____

Evening _____

New Foods/Reactions: _____

Stools (amount, number and type): _____

_____

Quick Symptoms Checklist: **Rate Symptoms 0-10**

❑ Headache	❑ Digestive symptoms	Energy level:_____
❑ Joint pain	❑ Abdominal pain	Mood: _____
❑ Muscle pain	❑ Tinnitus	Mental Clarity: _____
❑ Other: _____	❑ Other: _____	Purpose/Hope: _____

Date _____

❏ FCLO/HVBO	❏ Probiotic	❏ Detox Bath	❏ AM Juicing	❏ Fat
❏ Omega 3/6	❏ Beet Kvass	❏ Oil Pull	❏ PM Juicing	❏ Stock
❏ Iodine	❏ Milk Kefir	❏ Sunbathing	❏ Movement	❏ Ferments

Take a Moment:

Learning is a treasure that will follow its owner everywhere.
—Chinese Proverb

Learn something today. Write it here.

_____

_____

_____

Today's Focus: _____

Nutritional Intake:

Breakfast _____

Mid-morning_____

Lunch _____

Mid-afternoon _____

Dinner _____

Evening _____

New Foods/Reactions:_____

Stools (amount, number and type): _____

_____

Quick Symptoms Checklist:		**Rate Symptoms 0-10**
❏ Headache	❏ Digestive symptoms	Energy level:_____
❏ Joint pain	❏ Abdominal pain	Mood: _____
❏ Muscle pain	❏ Tinnitus	Mental Clarity: _____
❏ Other: _____	❏ Other: _____	Purpose/Hope: _____

Date _____

❏ FCLO/HVBO	❏ Probiotic	❏ Detox Bath	❏ AM Juicing	❏ Fat
❏ Omega 3/6	❏ Beet Kvass	❏ Oil Pull	❏ PM Juicing	❏ Stock
❏ Iodine	❏ Milk Kefir	❏ Sunbathing	❏ Movement	❏ Ferments

Take a Moment:

I am seeking. I am striving. I am in it with all my heart.
—Vincent Van Gogh

What are you seeking and striving toward?

_____

_____

_____

Today's Focus: _____

Nutritional Intake:

Breakfast _____

Mid-morning _____

Lunch _____

Mid-afternoon _____

Dinner _____

Evening _____

New Foods/Reactions: _____

Stools (amount, number and type): _____

_____

Quick Symptoms Checklist: **Rate Symptoms 0-10**

❏ Headache	❏ Digestive symptoms	Energy level:_____
❏ Joint pain	❏ Abdominal pain	Mood: _____
❏ Muscle pain	❏ Tinnitus	Mental Clarity:_____
❏ Other: _____	❏ Other: _____	Purpose/Hope: _____

Date _____

❏ FCLO/HVBO	❏ Probiotic	❏ Detox Bath	❏ AM Juicing	❏ Fat
❏ Omega 3/6	❏ Beet Kvass	❏ Oil Pull	❏ PM Juicing	❏ Stock
❏ Iodine	❏ Milk Kefir	❏ Sunbathing	❏ Movement	❏ Ferments

Take a Moment:

> *To become different from what we are, we must have some awareness of what we are.* —Eric Hoffer

Take some time today to think about what you are.

_____

_____

_____

Today's Focus: _____

Nutritional Intake:

Breakfast _____

Mid-morning_____

Lunch _____

Mid-afternoon _____

Dinner _____

Evening _____

New Foods/Reactions:_____

Stools (amount, number and type): _____

_____

Quick Symptoms Checklist: **Rate Symptoms 0-10**

❏ Headache	❏ Digestive symptoms	Energy level:_____
❏ Joint pain	❏ Abdominal pain	Mood: _____
❏ Muscle pain	❏ Tinnitus	Mental Clarity: _____
❏ Other: _____	❏ Other: _____	Purpose/Hope: _____

My week overall: 0--10

I would describe my week (in one word) as: _____

Because? _____

General progress:

Advanced to a new stage? Y/N   Current stage?_____

New foods tolerated: _____   Foods removed: _____

Animal fats consumed: _____   Avg. daily amount: _____

# of days stock consumed: _____   Avg. daily amount: _____

Probiotics/fermented foods/cultured dairy:

Probiotic supplement: _____Current dose: _____

Die-off symptoms: Y/N   Describe: _____

_____

Beet Kvass _____   Sour Cream _____

Veggie Medley_____   Yogurt _____

Sauerkraut_____   Kefir_____

Detoxing Progress:

# of detox baths: _____ Ingredients: ACV/Epsom/Baking soda

# of days sunbathed: _____ # of minutes per session:_____ minutes

# of days juiced in am: _____in pm: _____

Ingredients:_____

Overall reactions to detoxing: _____

Symptoms descriptions:

Stools: Daily Y/N   #per day _____   Type(s):_____

Digestion: _____

Mood/energy: _____

Memory/clarity: _____

Sleep/Stress: _____

Typical-for-me symptoms: _____

_____

Date _____

❏ FCLO/HVBO	❏ Probiotic	❏ Detox Bath	❏ AM Juicing	❏ Fat
❏ Omega 3/6	❏ Beet Kvass	❏ Oil Pull	❏ PM Juicing	❏ Stock
❏ Iodine	❏ Milk Kefir	❏ Sunbathing	❏ Movement	❏ Ferments

Take a Moment:

Where there is no vision, there is no hope. —George Washington Carver

Are you low on hope? Write about your vision.

_____

_____

_____

_____

Today's Focus: _____

Nutritional Intake:

Breakfast _____

Mid-morning _____

Lunch _____

Mid-afternoon _____

Dinner _____

Evening _____

New Foods/Reactions: _____

Stools (amount, number and type): _____

Quick Symptoms Checklist: Rate Symptoms 0-10

❏ Headache	❏ Digestive symptoms	Energy level:_____
❏ Joint pain	❏ Abdominal pain	Mood: _____
❏ Muscle pain	❏ Tinnitus	Mental Clarity: _____
❏ Other: _____	❏ Other: _____	Purpose/Hope: _____

Date _____

❏ FCLO/HVBO	❏ Probiotic	❏ Detox Bath	❏ AM Juicing	❏ Fat
❏ Omega 3/6	❏ Beet Kvass	❏ Oil Pull	❏ PM Juicing	❏ Stock
❏ Iodine	❏ Milk Kefir	❏ Sunbathing	❏ Movement	❏ Ferments

Take a Moment:

No duty is more urgent than that of returning thanks. —James Allen

What can you say thank you for today?

_____

_____

_____

_____

Today's Focus: _____

Nutritional Intake:

Breakfast _____

Mid-morning_____

Lunch _____

Mid-afternoon _____

Dinner _____

Evening _____

New Foods/Reactions: _____

Stools (amount, number and type): _____

_____

Quick Symptoms Checklist: **Rate Symptoms 0-10**

❏ Headache	❏ Digestive symptoms	Energy level:_____
❏ Joint pain	❏ Abdominal pain	Mood: _____
❏ Muscle pain	❏ Tinnitus	Mental Clarity:_____
❏ Other: _____	❏ Other: _____	Purpose/Hope: _____

Date _____

❑ FCLO/HVBO	❑ Probiotic	❑ Detox Bath	❑ AM Juicing	❑ Fat
❑ Omega 3/6	❑ Beet Kvass	❑ Oil Pull	❑ PM Juicing	❑ Stock
❑ Iodine	❑ Milk Kefir	❑ Sunbathing	❑ Movement	❑ Ferments

Take a Moment:

Go as far as you can see; when you get there, you'll be able to see farther. —J.P. Morgan

How far can you see? Can you start going that far?

_____

_____

_____

Today's Focus: _____

Nutritional Intake:

Breakfast _____

Mid-morning_____

Lunch _____

Mid-afternoon _____

Dinner _____

Evening _____

New Foods/Reactions: _____

Stools (amount, number and type): _____

_____

Quick Symptoms Checklist:		**Rate Symptoms 0-10**
❑ Headache	❑ Digestive symptoms	Energy level:_____
❑ Joint pain	❑ Abdominal pain	Mood: _____
❑ Muscle pain	❑ Tinnitus	Mental Clarity: _____
❑ Other: _____	❑ Other: _____	Purpose/Hope: _____

Date _____

❑ FCLO/HVBO	❑ Probiotic	❑ Detox Bath	❑ AM Juicing	❑ Fat
❑ Omega 3/6	❑ Beet Kvass	❑ Oil Pull	❑ PM Juicing	❑ Stock
❑ Iodine	❑ Milk Kefir	❑ Sunbathing	❑ Movement	❑ Ferments

Take a Moment:

There is only one corner of the universe you can be certain of improving, and that's your own self. —Aldous Huxley

It can be frustrating to see how people around you could change for the better. You can only control you. What do you need to let go of?

_____

_____

_____

Today's Focus: _____

Nutritional Intake:

Breakfast _____

Mid-morning _____

Lunch _____

Mid-afternoon _____

Dinner _____

Evening _____

New Foods/Reactions: _____

Stools (amount, number and type): _____

_____

Quick Symptoms Checklist:		**Rate Symptoms 0-10**
❑ Headache	❑ Digestive symptoms	Energy level:_____
❑ Joint pain	❑ Abdominal pain	Mood: _____
❑ Muscle pain	❑ Tinnitus	Mental Clarity:_____
❑ Other: _____	❑ Other: _____	Purpose/Hope: _____

Date _____

❑ FCLO/HVBO	❑ Probiotic	❑ Detox Bath	❑ AM Juicing	❑ Fat
❑ Omega 3/6	❑ Beet Kvass	❑ Oil Pull	❑ PM Juicing	❑ Stock
❑ Iodine	❑ Milk Kefir	❑ Sunbathing	❑ Movement	❑ Ferments

Take a Moment:

Early to bed and early to rise, makes a man healthy, wealthy, and wise.
—Benjamin Franklin

Get a good start to your week. Make a plan to get to bed earlier tonight.

_____

_____

_____

Today's Focus: _____

Nutritional Intake:

Breakfast _____

Mid-morning_____

Lunch _____

Mid-afternoon _____

Dinner _____

Evening _____

New Foods/Reactions: _____

Stools (amount, number and type): _____

Quick Symptoms Checklist: **Rate Symptoms 0-10**

❑ Headache	❑ Digestive symptoms	Energy level:_____
❑ Joint pain	❑ Abdominal pain	Mood: _____
❑ Muscle pain	❑ Tinnitus	Mental Clarity: _____
❑ Other: _____	❑ Other: _____	Purpose/Hope: _____

Date _____

❑ FCLO/HVBO	❑ Probiotic	❑ Detox Bath	❑ AM Juicing	❑ Fat
❑ Omega 3/6	❑ Beet Kvass	❑ Oil Pull	❑ PM Juicing	❑ Stock
❑ Iodine	❑ Milk Kefir	❑ Sunbathing	❑ Movement	❑ Ferments

Take a Moment:

There are as many nights as days, and the one is just as long as the other in the year's course. Even a happy life cannot be without a measure of darkness, and the word happy would lose its meaning if it were not balanced by sadness. —Carl Gustav Jung

How has "happy" been defined by sadness in your life?

_____

_____

Today's Focus: _____

Nutritional Intake:

Breakfast _____

Mid-morning_____

Lunch _____

Mid-afternoon _____

Dinner _____

Evening _____

New Foods/Reactions: _____

Stools (amount, number and type): _____

Quick Symptoms Checklist: | **Rate Symptoms 0-10**

❑ Headache	❑ Digestive symptoms	Energy level:_____
❑ Joint pain	❑ Abdominal pain	Mood: _____
❑ Muscle pain	❑ Tinnitus	Mental Clarity: _____
❑ Other: _____	❑ Other: _____	Purpose/Hope: _____

Date _____

❑ FCLO/HVBO	❑ Probiotic	❑ Detox Bath	❑ AM Juicing	❑ Fat
❑ Omega 3/6	❑ Beet Kvass	❑ Oil Pull	❑ PM Juicing	❑ Stock
❑ Iodine	❑ Milk Kefir	❑ Sunbathing	❑ Movement	❑ Ferments

Take a Moment:

> *Whenever you take a step forward, you are bound to disturb something.* —Indria Gandhi

Think back over what you have disturbed in the last couple months. What forward steps does that represent?

_____

_____

Today's Focus: _____

Nutritional Intake:

Breakfast _____

Mid-morning_____

Lunch _____

Mid-afternoon _____

Dinner _____

Evening _____

New Foods/Reactions: _____

Stools (amount, number and type): _____

_____

Quick Symptoms Checklist: **Rate Symptoms 0-10**

❑ Headache	❑ Digestive symptoms	Energy level:_____
❑ Joint pain	❑ Abdominal pain	Mood: _____
❑ Muscle pain	❑ Tinnitus	Mental Clarity:_____
❑ Other: _____	❑ Other: _____	Purpose/Hope: _____

My week overall: 0--10

I would describe my week (in one word) as: _____

Because? _____

General progress:

Advanced to a new stage? Y/N   Current stage?_____

New foods tolerated: _____   Foods removed: _____

Animal fats consumed: _____   Avg. daily amount: _____

# of days stock consumed: _____   Avg. daily amount: _____

Probiotics/fermented foods/cultured dairy:

Probiotic supplement: _____Current dose: _____

Die-off symptoms: Y/N   Describe: _____

_____

Beet Kvass _____   Sour Cream _____

Veggie Medley_____   Yogurt _____

Sauerkraut_____   Kefir_____

Detoxing Progress:

# of detox baths: _____ Ingredients: ACV/Epsom/Baking soda

# of days sunbathed: _____ # of minutes per session:_____ minutes

# of days juiced in am: _____in pm: _____

Ingredients:_____

Overall reactions to detoxing: _____

Symptoms descriptions:

Stools: Daily Y/N   #per day _____   Type(s):_____

Digestion: _____

Mood/energy: _____

Memory/clarity: _____

Sleep/Stress: _____

Typical-for-me symptoms: _____

_____

Date _____

❏ FCLO/HVBO	❏ Probiotic	❏ Detox Bath	❏ AM Juicing	❏ Fat
❏ Omega 3/6	❏ Beet Kvass	❏ Oil Pull	❏ PM Juicing	❏ Stock
❏ Iodine	❏ Milk Kefir	❏ Sunbathing	❏ Movement	❏ Ferments

Take a Moment:

Here is a test to find out whether your mission on earth is finished: If you are alive, it isn't. —Richard Bach

Do you believe that you still have a purpose to be here?

_____

_____

_____

Today's Focus: _____

Nutritional Intake:

Breakfast _____

Mid-morning_____

Lunch _____

Mid-afternoon _____

Dinner _____

Evening _____

New Foods/Reactions: _____

Stools (amount, number and type): _____

Quick Symptoms Checklist: **Rate Symptoms 0-10**

❏ Headache	❏ Digestive symptoms	Energy level:_____
❏ Joint pain	❏ Abdominal pain	Mood: _____
❏ Muscle pain	❏ Tinnitus	Mental Clarity: _____
❏ Other: _____	❏ Other: _____	Purpose/Hope: _____

Date _____

❑ FCLO/HVBO	❑ Probiotic	❑ Detox Bath	❑ AM Juicing	❑ Fat
❑ Omega 3/6	❑ Beet Kvass	❑ Oil Pull	❑ PM Juicing	❑ Stock
❑ Iodine	❑ Milk Kefir	❑ Sunbathing	❑ Movement	❑ Ferments

Take a Moment:

Courage is doing what you're afraid to do. There can be no courage unless you're scared. —Eddie Rickenbacker

Do you believe you have courage, especially when you're scared?

_____

_____

_____

Today's Focus: _____

Nutritional Intake:

Breakfast _____

Mid-morning_____

Lunch _____

Mid-afternoon _____

Dinner _____

Evening _____

New Foods/Reactions: _____

Stools (amount, number and type): _____

Quick Symptoms Checklist: **Rate Symptoms 0-10**

❑ Headache	❑ Digestive symptoms	Energy level:_____
❑ Joint pain	❑ Abdominal pain	Mood: _____
❑ Muscle pain	❑ Tinnitus	Mental Clarity: _____
❑ Other: _____	❑ Other: _____	Purpose/Hope: _____

❑ FCLO/HVBO	❑ Probiotic	❑ Detox Bath	❑ AM Juicing	❑ Fat
❑ Omega 3/6	❑ Beet Kvass	❑ Oil Pull	❑ PM Juicing	❑ Stock
❑ Iodine	❑ Milk Kefir	❑ Sunbathing	❑ Movement	❑ Ferments

Take a Moment:

A problem is a chance for you to do your best. —Duke Ellington

What problem are you facing today?

_____

_____

_____

_____

Today's Focus: _____

Nutritional Intake:

Breakfast _____

Mid-morning_____

Lunch _____

Mid-afternoon _____

Dinner _____

Evening _____

New Foods/Reactions:_____

Stools (amount, number and type): _____

Quick Symptoms Checklist: **Rate Symptoms 0-10**

❑ Headache	❑ Digestive symptoms	Energy level:_____
❑ Joint pain	❑ Abdominal pain	Mood: _____
❑ Muscle pain	❑ Tinnitus	Mental Clarity: _____
❑ Other: _____	❑ Other: _____	Purpose/Hope: _____

❑ FCLO/HVBO	❑ Probiotic	❑ Detox Bath	❑ AM Juicing	❑ Fat
❑ Omega 3/6	❑ Beet Kvass	❑ Oil Pull	❑ PM Juicing	❑ Stock
❑ Iodine	❑ Milk Kefir	❑ Sunbathing	❑ Movement	❑ Ferments

Take a Moment:

Laughter is the shortest distance between two people. —Victor Borge

It's not always easy to laugh. Tell how you were able to laugh today.

_____

_____

_____

_____

Today's Focus: _____

Nutritional Intake:

Breakfast _____

Mid-morning_____

Lunch _____

Mid-afternoon _____

Dinner _____

Evening _____

New Foods/Reactions: _____

Stools (amount, number and type): _____

Quick Symptoms Checklist:		Rate Symptoms 0-10
❑ Headache	❑ Digestive symptoms	Energy level:_____
❑ Joint pain	❑ Abdominal pain	Mood: _____
❑ Muscle pain	❑ Tinnitus	Mental Clarity:_____
❑ Other: _____	❑ Other: _____	Purpose/Hope: _____

Date _____

❏ FCLO/HVBO	❏ Probiotic	❏ Detox Bath	❏ AM Juicing	❏ Fat
❏ Omega 3/6	❏ Beet Kvass	❏ Oil Pull	❏ PM Juicing	❏ Stock
❏ Iodine	❏ Milk Kefir	❏ Sunbathing	❏ Movement	❏ Ferments

Take a Moment:

Never give up on a dream just because of the time it will take to accomplish it. The time will pass anyway. —Earl Nightengale

Do you want to give up?

_____

_____

_____

Today's Focus: _____

Nutritional Intake:

Breakfast _____

Mid-morning_____

Lunch _____

Mid-afternoon _____

Dinner _____

Evening _____

New Foods/Reactions: _____

Stools (amount, number and type): _____

Quick Symptoms Checklist:		Rate Symptoms 0-10
❏ Headache	❏ Digestive symptoms	Energy level:_____
❏ Joint pain	❏ Abdominal pain	Mood: _____
❏ Muscle pain	❏ Tinnitus	Mental Clarity: _____
❏ Other: _____	❏ Other: _____	Purpose/Hope: _____

Date _____

❑ FCLO/HVBO	❑ Probiotic	❑ Detox Bath	❑ AM Juicing	❑ Fat
❑ Omega 3/6	❑ Beet Kvass	❑ Oil Pull	❑ PM Juicing	❑ Stock
❑ Iodine	❑ Milk Kefir	❑ Sunbathing	❑ Movement	❑ Ferments

Take a Moment:

Adversity draws men together and produces beauty and harmony in life's relationships, just as the cold of winter produces ice-flowers on the windowpanes, which vanish with the warmth. —Søren Kierkegaard

What beauty is adversity producing in you?

_____

_____

_____

Today's Focus: _____

Nutritional Intake:

Breakfast _____

Mid-morning _____

Lunch _____

Mid-afternoon _____

Dinner _____

Evening _____

New Foods/Reactions: _____

Stools (amount, number and type): _____

_____

Quick Symptoms Checklist: Rate Symptoms 0-10

❑ Headache	❑ Digestive symptoms	Energy level:_____
❑ Joint pain	❑ Abdominal pain	Mood: _____
❑ Muscle pain	❑ Tinnitus	Mental Clarity:_____
❑ Other: _____	❑ Other: _____	Purpose/Hope: _____

Date _____

❑ FCLO/HVBO	❑ Probiotic	❑ Detox Bath	❑ AM Juicing	❑ Fat
❑ Omega 3/6	❑ Beet Kvass	❑ Oil Pull	❑ PM Juicing	❑ Stock
❑ Iodine	❑ Milk Kefir	❑ Sunbathing	❑ Movement	❑ Ferments

Take a Moment:

Peace begins with a smile. —Mother Teresa

Start your day with a smile. Does a smile bring you peace?

_____

_____

_____

_____

Today's Focus: _____

Nutritional Intake:

Breakfast _____

Mid-morning _____

Lunch _____

Mid-afternoon _____

Dinner _____

Evening _____

New Foods/Reactions: _____

Stools (amount, number and type): _____

_____

Quick Symptoms Checklist:		Rate Symptoms 0-10
❑ Headache	❑ Digestive symptoms	Energy level: _____
❑ Joint pain	❑ Abdominal pain	Mood: _____
❑ Muscle pain	❑ Tinnitus	Mental Clarity: _____
❑ Other: _____	❑ Other: _____	Purpose/Hope: _____

My week overall: 0--10

I would describe my week (in one word) as: _____

Because? _____

General progress:

Advanced to a new stage? Y/N   Current stage?_____

New foods tolerated: _____   Foods removed: _____

Animal fats consumed: _____   Avg. daily amount: _____

# of days stock consumed: _____   Avg. daily amount: _____

Probiotics/fermented foods/cultured dairy:

Probiotic supplement: _____Current dose: _____

Die-off symptoms: Y/N   Describe: _____

_____

Beet Kvass _____   Sour Cream _____

Veggie Medley_____   Yogurt _____

Sauerkraut_____   Kefir_____

Detoxing Progress:

# of detox baths: _____ Ingredients: ACV/Epsom/Baking soda

# of days sunbathed: _____ # of minutes per session:_____ minutes

# of days juiced in am: _____in pm: _____

Ingredients:_____

Overall reactions to detoxing: _____

Symptoms descriptions:

Stools: Daily Y/N   #per day _____   Type(s):_____

Digestion: _____

Mood/energy: _____

Memory/clarity: _____

Sleep/Stress: _____

Typical-for-me symptoms: _____

_____

Date _____

❏ FCLO/HVBO	❏ Probiotic	❏ Detox Bath	❏ AM Juicing	❏ Fat
❏ Omega 3/6	❏ Beet Kvass	❏ Oil Pull	❏ PM Juicing	❏ Stock
❏ Iodine	❏ Milk Kefir	❏ Sunbathing	❏ Movement	❏ Ferments

Take a Moment:

The truth is that our finest moments are most likely to occur when we are feeling deeply uncomfortable, unhappy, or unfulfilled. For it is only in such moments, propelled by our discomfort, that we are likely to step out of our ruts and start searching for different ways or truer answers. —M. Scott Peck

Most likely you are doing GAPS because of discomfort. Is there another rut you are being compelled out of right now?

_____

_____

Today's Focus: _____

Nutritional Intake:

Breakfast _____

Mid-morning_____

Lunch _____

Mid-afternoon _____

Dinner _____

Evening _____

New Foods/Reactions: _____

Stools (amount, number and type): _____

_____

Quick Symptoms Checklist: Rate Symptoms 0-10

❏ Headache	❏ Digestive symptoms	Energy level:_____
❏ Joint pain	❏ Abdominal pain	Mood: _____
❏ Muscle pain	❏ Tinnitus	Mental Clarity: _____
❏ Other: _____	❏ Other: _____	Purpose/Hope: _____

Date _____

❏ FCLO/HVBO	❏ Probiotic	❏ Detox Bath	❏ AM Juicing	❏ Fat
❏ Omega 3/6	❏ Beet Kvass	❏ Oil Pull	❏ PM Juicing	❏ Stock
❏ Iodine	❏ Milk Kefir	❏ Sunbathing	❏ Movement	❏ Ferments

Take a Moment:

A sense of humor is part of the art of leadership, of getting along with people, of getting things done. —Dwight D. Eisenhower

How is your sense of humor? Can it grow?

_____

_____

_____

Today's Focus: _____

Nutritional Intake:

Breakfast _____

Mid-morning _____

Lunch _____

Mid-afternoon _____

Dinner _____

Evening _____

New Foods/Reactions: _____

Stools (amount, number and type): _____

_____

Quick Symptoms Checklist: **Rate Symptoms 0-10**

❏ Headache	❏ Digestive symptoms	Energy level:_____
❏ Joint pain	❏ Abdominal pain	Mood: _____
❏ Muscle pain	❏ Tinnitus	Mental Clarity: _____
❏ Other: _____	❏ Other: _____	Purpose/Hope: _____

Date _____

❏ FCLO/HVBO	❏ Probiotic	❏ Detox Bath	❏ AM Juicing	❏ Fat
❏ Omega 3/6	❏ Beet Kvass	❏ Oil Pull	❏ PM Juicing	❏ Stock
❏ Iodine	❏ Milk Kefir	❏ Sunbathing	❏ Movement	❏ Ferments

Take a Moment:

The 'how' thinker gets problems solved effectively because he wastes no time with futile 'ifs'. —Norman Vincent Peale

What problem are you stuck on because you are bogged down in 'ifs'?

_____

_____

_____

Today's Focus: _____

Nutritional Intake:

Breakfast _____

Mid-morning_____

Lunch _____

Mid-afternoon _____

Dinner _____

Evening _____

New Foods/Reactions:_____

Stools (amount, number and type): _____

_____

Quick Symptoms Checklist: **Rate Symptoms 0-10**

❏ Headache	❏ Digestive symptoms	Energy level:_____
❏ Joint pain	❏ Abdominal pain	Mood: _____
❏ Muscle pain	❏ Tinnitus	Mental Clarity: _____
❏ Other: _____	❏ Other: _____	Purpose/Hope: _____

Date _____

❏ FCLO/HVBO	❏ Probiotic	❏ Detox Bath	❏ AM Juicing	❏ Fat
❏ Omega 3/6	❏ Beet Kvass	❏ Oil Pull	❏ PM Juicing	❏ Stock
❏ Iodine	❏ Milk Kefir	❏ Sunbathing	❏ Movement	❏ Ferments

Take a Moment:

Sometimes your joy is the source of your smile, but sometimes your smile can be the source of your joy. —Thich Nhat Hanh

Our minds are powerful. Write down at least one thought that can make you smile today, then think about it.

_____

_____

_____

Today's Focus: _____

Nutritional Intake:

Breakfast _____

Mid-morning_____

Lunch _____

Mid-afternoon _____

Dinner _____

Evening _____

New Foods/Reactions:_____

Stools (amount, number and type): _____

_____

Quick Symptoms Checklist: Rate Symptoms 0-10

❏ Headache	❏ Digestive symptoms	Energy level:_____
❏ Joint pain	❏ Abdominal pain	Mood: _____
❏ Muscle pain	❏ Tinnitus	Mental Clarity:_____
❏ Other: _____	❏ Other: _____	Purpose/Hope: _____

Date _____

❑ FCLO/HVBO	❑ Probiotic	❑ Detox Bath	❑ AM Juicing	❑ Fat
❑ Omega 3/6	❑ Beet Kvass	❑ Oil Pull	❑ PM Juicing	❑ Stock
❑ Iodine	❑ Milk Kefir	❑ Sunbathing	❑ Movement	❑ Ferments

Take a Moment:

What it lies in our power to do, it lies in our power not to do. —Aristotle

What is in your power to do? Are you going to do it today?

_____

_____

_____

_____

Today's Focus: _____

Nutritional Intake:

Breakfast _____

Mid-morning_____

Lunch _____

Mid-afternoon _____

Dinner _____

Evening _____

New Foods/Reactions: _____

Stools (amount, number and type): _____

_____

Quick Symptoms Checklist: **Rate Symptoms 0-10**

❑ Headache	❑ Digestive symptoms	Energy level:_____
❑ Joint pain	❑ Abdominal pain	Mood: _____
❑ Muscle pain	❑ Tinnitus	Mental Clarity: _____
❑ Other: _____	❑ Other: _____	Purpose/Hope: _____

Date _____

❏ FCLO/HVBO	❏ Probiotic	❏ Detox Bath	❏ AM Juicing	❏ Fat
❏ Omega 3/6	❏ Beet Kvass	❏ Oil Pull	❏ PM Juicing	❏ Stock
❏ Iodine	❏ Milk Kefir	❏ Sunbathing	❏ Movement	❏ Ferments

Take a Moment:

A helping word to one in trouble is often like a switch in a railroad track . . . an inch between a wreck and smooth, rolling prosperity.
—Henry Ward Beecher

Has someone given a helping word to you recently? What was it?

_____

_____

_____

Today's Focus: _____

Nutritional Intake:

Breakfast _____

Mid-morning_____

Lunch _____

Mid-afternoon _____

Dinner _____

Evening _____

New Foods/Reactions: _____

Stools (amount, number and type): _____

_____

Quick Symptoms Checklist: Rate Symptoms 0-10

❏ Headache	❏ Digestive symptoms	Energy level:_____
❏ Joint pain	❏ Abdominal pain	Mood: _____
❏ Muscle pain	❏ Tinnitus	Mental Clarity: _____
❏ Other: _____	❏ Other: _____	Purpose/Hope: _____

Date _____

❏ FCLO/HVBO	❏ Probiotic	❏ Detox Bath	❏ AM Juicing	❏ Fat
❏ Omega 3/6	❏ Beet Kvass	❏ Oil Pull	❏ PM Juicing	❏ Stock
❏ Iodine	❏ Milk Kefir	❏ Sunbathing	❏ Movement	❏ Ferments

Take a Moment:

A human being has a natural desire to have more of a good thing than he needs. —Mark Twain

Have you experienced this? What was the outcome for you?

_____

_____

_____

Today's Focus: _____

Nutritional Intake:

Breakfast _____

Mid-morning _____

Lunch _____

Mid-afternoon _____

Dinner _____

Evening _____

New Foods/Reactions: _____

Stools (amount, number and type): _____

Quick Symptoms Checklist: **Rate Symptoms 0-10**

❏ Headache	❏ Digestive symptoms	Energy level: _____
❏ Joint pain	❏ Abdominal pain	Mood: _____
❏ Muscle pain	❏ Tinnitus	Mental Clarity: _____
❏ Other: _____	❏ Other: _____	Purpose/Hope: _____

My week overall: 0--10

I would describe my week (in one word) as: _____

Because? _____

General progress:

Advanced to a new stage? Y/N   Current stage?_____

New foods tolerated: _____   Foods removed: _____

Animal fats consumed: _____   Avg. daily amount: _____

# of days stock consumed: _____   Avg. daily amount: _____

Probiotics/fermented foods/cultured dairy:

Probiotic supplement: _____Current dose: _____

Die-off symptoms: Y/N   Describe: _____

_____

Beet Kvass _____   Sour Cream _____

Veggie Medley _____   Yogurt _____

Sauerkraut_____   Kefir_____

Detoxing Progress:

# of detox baths: _____ Ingredients: ACV/Epsom/Baking soda

# of days sunbathed: _____ # of minutes per session:_____ minutes

# of days juiced in am: _____in pm: _____

Ingredients:_____

Overall reactions to detoxing: _____

Symptoms descriptions:

Stools: Daily Y/N   #per day _____   Type(s):_____

Digestion: _____

Mood/energy: _____

Memory/clarity: _____

Sleep/Stress: _____

Typical-for-me symptoms: _____

_____

Date _____

❏ FCLO/HVBO	❏ Probiotic	❏ Detox Bath	❏ AM Juicing	❏ Fat
❏ Omega 3/6	❏ Beet Kvass	❏ Oil Pull	❏ PM Juicing	❏ Stock
❏ Iodine	❏ Milk Kefir	❏ Sunbathing	❏ Movement	❏ Ferments

Take a Moment:

> *They say that time changes things, but you actually have
> to change them yourself.* —Andy Warhol

What have you been waiting for time to change, that you could actually work on yourself?

_____

_____

_____

Today's Focus: _____

Nutritional Intake:

Breakfast _____

Mid-morning _____

Lunch _____

Mid-afternoon _____

Dinner _____

Evening _____

New Foods/Reactions: _____

Stools (amount, number and type): _____

Quick Symptoms Checklist:		Rate Symptoms 0-10
❏ Headache	❏ Digestive symptoms	Energy level:_____
❏ Joint pain	❏ Abdominal pain	Mood: _____
❏ Muscle pain	❏ Tinnitus	Mental Clarity:_____
❏ Other: _____	❏ Other: _____	Purpose/Hope: _____

Date _____

❏ FCLO/HVBO	❏ Probiotic	❏ Detox Bath	❏ AM Juicing	❏ Fat
❏ Omega 3/6	❏ Beet Kvass	❏ Oil Pull	❏ PM Juicing	❏ Stock
❏ Iodine	❏ Milk Kefir	❏ Sunbathing	❏ Movement	❏ Ferments

Take a Moment:

Firelight will not let you read fine stories, but it's warm and you won't see the dust on the floor. —Irish Proverb

What is somthing that you usually think negatively about?
Now think of some positives it brings to your life.

_____

_____

_____

Today's Focus: _____

Nutritional Intake:

Breakfast _____

Mid-morning_____

Lunch _____

Mid-afternoon _____

Dinner _____

Evening _____

New Foods/Reactions: _____

Stools (amount, number and type): _____

_____

Quick Symptoms Checklist: Rate Symptoms 0-10

❏ Headache	❏ Digestive symptoms	Energy level:_____
❏ Joint pain	❏ Abdominal pain	Mood: _____
❏ Muscle pain	❏ Tinnitus	Mental Clarity:_____
❏ Other: _____	❏ Other: _____	Purpose/Hope: _____

Date _____

❏ FCLO/HVBO	❏ Probiotic	❏ Detox Bath	❏ AM Juicing	❏ Fat
❏ Omega 3/6	❏ Beet Kvass	❏ Oil Pull	❏ PM Juicing	❏ Stock
❏ Iodine	❏ Milk Kefir	❏ Sunbathing	❏ Movement	❏ Ferments

Take a Moment:

Write it on your heart that every day is the best day in the year.
—Ralph Waldo Emerson

How is today the best day in the year?

_____

_____

_____

Today's Focus: _____

Nutritional Intake:

Breakfast _____

Mid-morning_____

Lunch _____

Mid-afternoon _____

Dinner _____

Evening _____

New Foods/Reactions: _____

Stools (amount, number and type): _____

Quick Symptoms Checklist: **Rate Symptoms 0-10**

❏ Headache	❏ Digestive symptoms	Energy level:_____
❏ Joint pain	❏ Abdominal pain	Mood: _____
❏ Muscle pain	❏ Tinnitus	Mental Clarity: _____
❏ Other: _____	❏ Other: _____	Purpose/Hope: _____

Date _____

❏ FCLO/HVBO	❏ Probiotic	❏ Detox Bath	❏ AM Juicing	❏ Fat
❏ Omega 3/6	❏ Beet Kvass	❏ Oil Pull	❏ PM Juicing	❏ Stock
❏ Iodine	❏ Milk Kefir	❏ Sunbathing	❏ Movement	❏ Ferments

Take a Moment:

Give me six hours to chop down a tree and I will spend the first four sharpening the ax. —Abraham Lincoln

Do you have a big job coming up? How can you prepare?

_____

_____

_____

Today's Focus: _____

Nutritional Intake:

Breakfast _____

Mid-morning_____

Lunch _____

Mid-afternoon _____

Dinner _____

Evening _____

New Foods/Reactions: _____

Stools (amount, number and type): _____

Quick Symptoms Checklist: **Rate Symptoms 0-10**

❏ Headache	❏ Digestive symptoms	Energy level:_____
❏ Joint pain	❏ Abdominal pain	Mood: _____
❏ Muscle pain	❏ Tinnitus	Mental Clarity:_____
❏ Other: _____	❏ Other: _____	Purpose/Hope: _____

Date _____

❏ FCLO/HVBO	❏ Probiotic	❏ Detox Bath	❏ AM Juicing	❏ Fat
❏ Omega 3/6	❏ Beet Kvass	❏ Oil Pull	❏ PM Juicing	❏ Stock
❏ Iodine	❏ Milk Kefir	❏ Sunbathing	❏ Movement	❏ Ferments

Take a Moment:

Never cut a tree down in the wintertime. Never make a negative decision in the low time. Never make your most important decisions when you are in your worst moods. Wait. Be patient. The storm will pass. The spring will come.
—Robert H Schuller

Are you about to make a decision in a low time? Can you hang on a little and wait for spring?

_____

_____

Today's Focus: _____

Nutritional Intake:

Breakfast _____

Mid-morning_____

Lunch _____

Mid-afternoon _____

Dinner _____

Evening _____

New Foods/Reactions: _____

Stools (amount, number and type): _____

Quick Symptoms Checklist: | **Rate Symptoms 0-10**

❏ Headache	❏ Digestive symptoms	Energy level:_____
❏ Joint pain	❏ Abdominal pain	Mood: _____
❏ Muscle pain	❏ Tinnitus	Mental Clarity: _____
❏ Other: _____	❏ Other: _____	Purpose/Hope: _____

Date _____

❑ FCLO/HVBO	❑ Probiotic	❑ Detox Bath	❑ AM Juicing	❑ Fat
❑ Omega 3/6	❑ Beet Kvass	❑ Oil Pull	❑ PM Juicing	❑ Stock
❑ Iodine	❑ Milk Kefir	❑ Sunbathing	❑ Movement	❑ Ferments

Take a Moment:

Not truth, but faith it is that keeps the world alive. —Edna St. Vincent Millay

What faith keeps you going? Share this encouragement with someone else today.

_____

_____

_____

Today's Focus: _____

Nutritional Intake:

Breakfast _____

Mid-morning _____

Lunch _____

Mid-afternoon _____

Dinner _____

Evening _____

New Foods/Reactions: _____

Stools (amount, number and type): _____

Quick Symptoms Checklist: Rate Symptoms 0-10

❑ Headache	❑ Digestive symptoms	Energy level: _____
❑ Joint pain	❑ Abdominal pain	Mood: _____
❑ Muscle pain	❑ Tinnitus	Mental Clarity: _____
❑ Other: _____	❑ Other: _____	Purpose/Hope: _____

Date _____

❏ FCLO/HVBO	❏ Probiotic	❏ Detox Bath	❏ AM Juicing	❏ Fat
❏ Omega 3/6	❏ Beet Kvass	❏ Oil Pull	❏ PM Juicing	❏ Stock
❏ Iodine	❏ Milk Kefir	❏ Sunbathing	❏ Movement	❏ Ferments

Take a Moment:

*People grow through experience if they meet
life honestly and courageously.* —Eleanor Roosevelt

Do you meet life this way? Did you experience growth?

_____

_____

_____

Today's Focus: _____

Nutritional Intake:

Breakfast _____

Mid-morning _____

Lunch _____

Mid-afternoon _____

Dinner _____

Evening _____

New Foods/Reactions: _____

Stools (amount, number and type): _____

_____

Quick Symptoms Checklist:		**Rate Symptoms 0-10**
❏ Headache	❏ Digestive symptoms	Energy level:_____
❏ Joint pain	❏ Abdominal pain	Mood: _____
❏ Muscle pain	❏ Tinnitus	Mental Clarity: _____
❏ Other: _____	❏ Other: _____	Purpose/Hope: _____

My week overall: 0---10

I would describe my week (in one word) as: _____

Because? _____

General progress:

Advanced to a new stage? Y/N   Current stage?_____

New foods tolerated: _____   Foods removed: _____

Animal fats consumed: _____   Avg. daily amount: _____

# of days stock consumed: _____   Avg. daily amount: _____

Probiotics/fermented foods/cultured dairy:

Probiotic supplement: _____Current dose: _____

Die-off symptoms: Y/N   Describe: _____

_____

Beet Kvass _____   Sour Cream _____

Veggie Medley_____   Yogurt _____

Sauerkraut_____   Kefir_____

Detoxing Progress:

# of detox baths: _____ Ingredients: ACV/Epsom/Baking soda

# of days sunbathed: _____ # of minutes per session:_____ minutes

# of days juiced in am: _____in pm: _____

Ingredients:_____

Overall reactions to detoxing: _____

Symptoms descriptions:

Stools: Daily Y/N   #per day _____   Type(s):_____

Digestion: _____

Mood/energy: _____

Memory/clarity: _____

Sleep/Stress: _____

Typical-for-me symptoms: _____

_____

Date _____

❏ FCLO/HVBO	❏ Probiotic	❏ Detox Bath	❏ AM Juicing	❏ Fat
❏ Omega 3/6	❏ Beet Kvass	❏ Oil Pull	❏ PM Juicing	❏ Stock
❏ Iodine	❏ Milk Kefir	❏ Sunbathing	❏ Movement	❏ Ferments

Take a Moment:

> *If you don't like something, change it. If you can't change it,*
> *change your attitude.* —Maya Angelou

Think of something you can't change. Can you change your attitude?

_____

_____

_____

Today's Focus: _____

Nutritional Intake:

Breakfast _____

Mid-morning_____

Lunch _____

Mid-afternoon _____

Dinner _____

Evening _____

New Foods/Reactions:_____

Stools (amount, number and type): _____

Quick Symptoms Checklist: **Rate Symptoms 0-10**

❏ Headache	❏ Digestive symptoms	Energy level:_____
❏ Joint pain	❏ Abdominal pain	Mood: _____
❏ Muscle pain	❏ Tinnitus	Mental Clarity: _____
❏ Other: _____	❏ Other: _____	Purpose/Hope: _____

Date _____

❑ FCLO/HVBO	❑ Probiotic	❑ Detox Bath	❑ AM Juicing	❑ Fat
❑ Omega 3/6	❑ Beet Kvass	❑ Oil Pull	❑ PM Juicing	❑ Stock
❑ Iodine	❑ Milk Kefir	❑ Sunbathing	❑ Movement	❑ Ferments

Take a Moment:

Ever tried. Ever failed. No matter. Try again. Fail again. Fail better.
—Samuel Beckett

What is your motivation to try again today?

_____

_____

_____

Today's Focus: _____

Nutritional Intake:

Breakfast _____

Mid-morning_____

Lunch _____

Mid-afternoon _____

Dinner _____

Evening _____

New Foods/Reactions: _____

Stools (amount, number and type): _____

_____

Quick Symptoms Checklist: Rate Symptoms 0-10

❑ Headache	❑ Digestive symptoms	Energy level:_____
❑ Joint pain	❑ Abdominal pain	Mood: _____
❑ Muscle pain	❑ Tinnitus	Mental Clarity: _____
❑ Other: _____	❑ Other: _____	Purpose/Hope: _____

Date _____

❑ FCLO/HVBO	❑ Probiotic	❑ Detox Bath	❑ AM Juicing	❑ Fat
❑ Omega 3/6	❑ Beet Kvass	❑ Oil Pull	❑ PM Juicing	❑ Stock
❑ Iodine	❑ Milk Kefir	❑ Sunbathing	❑ Movement	❑ Ferments

Take a Moment:

Without a struggle, there can be no progress. —Frederick Douglass

What does your struggle feel like today?

_____

_____

_____

_____

Today's Focus: _____

Nutritional Intake:

Breakfast _____

Mid-morning _____

Lunch _____

Mid-afternoon _____

Dinner _____

Evening _____

New Foods/Reactions: _____

Stools (amount, number and type): _____

Quick Symptoms Checklist: **Rate Symptoms 0-10**

❑ Headache	❑ Digestive symptoms	Energy level:_____
❑ Joint pain	❑ Abdominal pain	Mood: _____
❑ Muscle pain	❑ Tinnitus	Mental Clarity: _____
❑ Other: _____	❑ Other: _____	Purpose/Hope: _____

Date _____

❏ FCLO/HVBO	❏ Probiotic	❏ Detox Bath	❏ AM Juicing	❏ Fat
❏ Omega 3/6	❏ Beet Kvass	❏ Oil Pull	❏ PM Juicing	❏ Stock
❏ Iodine	❏ Milk Kefir	❏ Sunbathing	❏ Movement	❏ Ferments

Take a Moment:

*She stood in the storm, and when the wind did not blow her way,
she adjusted her sails.* —Elizabeth Edwards

Do you need to make any adjustments in your sails?

_____

_____

_____

Today's Focus: _____

Nutritional Intake:

Breakfast _____

Mid-morning_____

Lunch _____

Mid-afternoon _____

Dinner _____

Evening _____

New Foods/Reactions:_____

Stools (amount, number and type): _____

Quick Symptoms Checklist: **Rate Symptoms 0-10**

❏ Headache	❏ Digestive symptoms	Energy level:_____
❏ Joint pain	❏ Abdominal pain	Mood: _____
❏ Muscle pain	❏ Tinnitus	Mental Clarity: _____
❏ Other: _____	❏ Other: _____	Purpose/Hope: _____

Date _____

❑ FCLO/HVBO	❑ Probiotic	❑ Detox Bath	❑ AM Juicing	❑ Fat
❑ Omega 3/6	❑ Beet Kvass	❑ Oil Pull	❑ PM Juicing	❑ Stock
❑ Iodine	❑ Milk Kefir	❑ Sunbathing	❑ Movement	❑ Ferments

Take a Moment:

Rock bottom became the solid foundation on which I rebuilt my life.
—J.K. Rowling

Do you feel like you have hit rock bottom? Write about how you are going to rebuild.

_____

_____

_____

Today's Focus: _____

Nutritional Intake:

Breakfast _____

Mid-morning_____

Lunch _____

Mid-afternoon _____

Dinner _____

Evening _____

New Foods/Reactions: _____

Stools (amount, number and type): _____

Quick Symptoms Checklist: Rate Symptoms 0-10

❑ Headache	❑ Digestive symptoms	Energy level:_____
❑ Joint pain	❑ Abdominal pain	Mood: _____
❑ Muscle pain	❑ Tinnitus	Mental Clarity: _____
❑ Other: _____	❑ Other: _____	Purpose/Hope: _____

Date _____

❑ FCLO/HVBO	❑ Probiotic	❑ Detox Bath	❑ AM Juicing	❑ Fat
❑ Omega 3/6	❑ Beet Kvass	❑ Oil Pull	❑ PM Juicing	❑ Stock
❑ Iodine	❑ Milk Kefir	❑ Sunbathing	❑ Movement	❑ Ferments

Take a Moment:

What does not destroy me, makes me stronger. —Friedrich Wilhelm Nietzsche

What has made you stronger?

_____

_____

_____

_____

Today's Focus: _____

Nutritional Intake:

Breakfast _____

Mid-morning_____

Lunch _____

Mid-afternoon _____

Dinner _____

Evening _____

New Foods/Reactions: _____

Stools (amount, number and type): _____

_____

Quick Symptoms Checklist: Rate Symptoms 0-10

❑ Headache	❑ Digestive symptoms	Energy level:_____
❑ Joint pain	❑ Abdominal pain	Mood: _____
❑ Muscle pain	❑ Tinnitus	Mental Clarity: _____
❑ Other: _____	❑ Other: _____	Purpose/Hope: _____

Date _____

❑ FCLO/HVBO	❑ Probiotic	❑ Detox Bath	❑ AM Juicing	❑ Fat
❑ Omega 3/6	❑ Beet Kvass	❑ Oil Pull	❑ PM Juicing	❑ Stock
❑ Iodine	❑ Milk Kefir	❑ Sunbathing	❑ Movement	❑ Ferments

Take a Moment:

> *If a man does not know what port he is steering for,*
> *no wind is favorable to him.* —Seneca

Take a moment to remind yourself what you are steering for.

_____

_____

_____

Today's Focus: _____

Nutritional Intake:

Breakfast _____

Mid-morning _____

Lunch _____

Mid-afternoon _____

Dinner _____

Evening _____

New Foods/Reactions: _____

Stools (amount, number and type): _____

Quick Symptoms Checklist: | **Rate Symptoms 0-10**

Quick Symptoms Checklist:		Rate Symptoms 0-10
❑ Headache	❑ Digestive symptoms	Energy level: _____
❑ Joint pain	❑ Abdominal pain	Mood: _____
❑ Muscle pain	❑ Tinnitus	Mental Clarity: _____
❑ Other: _____	❑ Other: _____	Purpose/Hope: _____

My week overall: 0---**10**

I would describe my week (in one word) as: _____

Because? _____

General progress:

Advanced to a new stage? Y/N   Current stage?_____

New foods tolerated: _____   Foods removed: _____

Animal fats consumed: _____   Avg. daily amount: _____

# of days stock consumed: _____   Avg. daily amount: _____

Probiotics/fermented foods/cultured dairy:

Probiotic supplement: _____Current dose: _____

Die-off symptoms: Y/N   Describe: _____

_____

Beet Kvass _____   Sour Cream _____

Veggie Medley_____   Yogurt _____

Sauerkraut_____   Kefir_____

Detoxing Progress:

# of detox baths: _____ Ingredients: ACV/Epsom/Baking soda

# of days sunbathed: _____ # of minutes per session:_____ minutes

# of days juiced in am: _____in pm: _____

Ingredients:_____

Overall reactions to detoxing: _____

Symptoms descriptions:

Stools: Daily Y/N   #per day _____   Type(s):_____

Digestion: _____

Mood/energy: _____

Memory/clarity: _____

Sleep/Stress: _____

Typical-for-me symptoms: _____

_____

Date _____

❏ FCLO/HVBO	❏ Probiotic	❏ Detox Bath	❏ AM Juicing	❏ Fat
❏ Omega 3/6	❏ Beet Kvass	❏ Oil Pull	❏ PM Juicing	❏ Stock
❏ Iodine	❏ Milk Kefir	❏ Sunbathing	❏ Movement	❏ Ferments

Take a Moment:

A man can get discouraged many times but he is not a failure until he begins to blame somebody else and stops trying. —John Burroughs

Are you blaming someone else? Are you still trying?

_____

_____

_____

Today's Focus: _____

Nutritional Intake:

Breakfast _____

Mid-morning_____

Lunch _____

Mid-afternoon _____

Dinner _____

Evening _____

New Foods/Reactions: _____

Stools (amount, number and type): _____

_____

Quick Symptoms Checklist:		**Rate Symptoms 0-10**
❏ Headache	❏ Digestive symptoms	Energy level:_____
❏ Joint pain	❏ Abdominal pain	Mood: _____
❏ Muscle pain	❏ Tinnitus	Mental Clarity: _____
❏ Other: _____	❏ Other: _____	Purpose/Hope: _____

Date _____

❏ FCLO/HVBO	❏ Probiotic	❏ Detox Bath	❏ AM Juicing	❏ Fat
❏ Omega 3/6	❏ Beet Kvass	❏ Oil Pull	❏ PM Juicing	❏ Stock
❏ Iodine	❏ Milk Kefir	❏ Sunbathing	❏ Movement	❏ Ferments

Take a Moment:

We cannot solve our problems with the same thinking we used when we created them. —Albert Einstein

Do you need to change your thinking in something?

_____

_____

_____

Today's Focus: _____

Nutritional Intake:

Breakfast _____

Mid-morning _____

Lunch _____

Mid-afternoon _____

Dinner _____

Evening _____

New Foods/Reactions: _____

Stools (amount, number and type): _____

_____

Quick Symptoms Checklist: **Rate Symptoms 0-10**

❏ Headache	❏ Digestive symptoms	Energy level:_____
❏ Joint pain	❏ Abdominal pain	Mood: _____
❏ Muscle pain	❏ Tinnitus	Mental Clarity:_____
❏ Other: _____	❏ Other: _____	Purpose/Hope: _____

Date _____

❏ FCLO/HVBO	❏ Probiotic	❏ Detox Bath	❏ AM Juicing	❏ Fat
❏ Omega 3/6	❏ Beet Kvass	❏ Oil Pull	❏ PM Juicing	❏ Stock
❏ Iodine	❏ Milk Kefir	❏ Sunbathing	❏ Movement	❏ Ferments

Take a Moment:

Anger can be an expensive luxury. —Italian Proverb

What does anger cost you?

_____

_____

_____

Today's Focus: _____

Nutritional Intake:

Breakfast _____

Mid-morning _____

Lunch _____

Mid-afternoon _____

Dinner _____

Evening _____

New Foods/Reactions: _____

Stools (amount, number and type): _____

_____

Quick Symptoms Checklist: **Rate Symptoms 0-10**

❏ Headache	❏ Digestive symptoms	Energy level: _____
❏ Joint pain	❏ Abdominal pain	Mood: _____
❏ Muscle pain	❏ Tinnitus	Mental Clarity: _____
❏ Other: _____	❏ Other: _____	Purpose/Hope: _____

Date _____

❑ FCLO/HVBO	❑ Probiotic	❑ Detox Bath	❑ AM Juicing	❑ Fat
❑ Omega 3/6	❑ Beet Kvass	❑ Oil Pull	❑ PM Juicing	❑ Stock
❑ Iodine	❑ Milk Kefir	❑ Sunbathing	❑ Movement	❑ Ferments

Take a Moment:

Life's most persistent and urgent question is,
'What are you doing for others?' —Martin Luther King, Jr.

What can you do for someone today?

_____

_____

_____

Today's Focus: _____

Nutritional Intake:

Breakfast _____

Mid-morning_____

Lunch _____

Mid-afternoon _____

Dinner _____

Evening _____

New Foods/Reactions: _____

Stools (amount, number and type): _____

Quick Symptoms Checklist: **Rate Symptoms 0-10**

❑ Headache	❑ Digestive symptoms	Energy level:_____
❑ Joint pain	❑ Abdominal pain	Mood: _____
❑ Muscle pain	❑ Tinnitus	Mental Clarity: _____
❑ Other: _____	❑ Other: _____	Purpose/Hope: _____

117

Date _____

❑ FCLO/HVBO	❑ Probiotic	❑ Detox Bath	❑ AM Juicing	❑ Fat
❑ Omega 3/6	❑ Beet Kvass	❑ Oil Pull	❑ PM Juicing	❑ Stock
❑ Iodine	❑ Milk Kefir	❑ Sunbathing	❑ Movement	❑ Ferments

Take a Moment:

Every day brings new choices. —Martha Beck

You will have choices today. How will you make them?

_____

_____

_____

_____

Today's Focus: _____

Nutritional Intake:

Breakfast _____

Mid-morning _____

Lunch _____

Mid-afternoon _____

Dinner _____

Evening _____

New Foods/Reactions: _____

Stools (amount, number and type): _____

Quick Symptoms Checklist: Rate Symptoms 0-10

❑ Headache	❑ Digestive symptoms	Energy level:_____
❑ Joint pain	❑ Abdominal pain	Mood: _____
❑ Muscle pain	❑ Tinnitus	Mental Clarity: _____
❑ Other: _____	❑ Other: _____	Purpose/Hope: _____

Date _____

❏ FCLO/HVBO	❏ Probiotic	❏ Detox Bath	❏ AM Juicing	❏ Fat
❏ Omega 3/6	❏ Beet Kvass	❏ Oil Pull	❏ PM Juicing	❏ Stock
❏ Iodine	❏ Milk Kefir	❏ Sunbathing	❏ Movement	❏ Ferments

Take a Moment:

In any moment of decision, the best thing you can do is the right thing, the next best thing is the wrong thing, and the worst thing you can do is nothing. —Theodore Roosevelt

Are you paralyzed by a decision?

_____

_____

_____

Today's Focus: _____

Nutritional Intake:

Breakfast _____

Mid-morning _____

Lunch _____

Mid-afternoon _____

Dinner _____

Evening _____

New Foods/Reactions: _____

Stools (amount, number and type): _____

Quick Symptoms Checklist: **Rate Symptoms 0-10**

❏ Headache	❏ Digestive symptoms	Energy level:_____
❏ Joint pain	❏ Abdominal pain	Mood: _____
❏ Muscle pain	❏ Tinnitus	Mental Clarity:_____
❏ Other: _____	❏ Other: _____	Purpose/Hope: _____

Date _____

❏ FCLO/HVBO	❏ Probiotic	❏ Detox Bath	❏ AM Juicing	❏ Fat
❏ Omega 3/6	❏ Beet Kvass	❏ Oil Pull	❏ PM Juicing	❏ Stock
❏ Iodine	❏ Milk Kefir	❏ Sunbathing	❏ Movement	❏ Ferments

Take a Moment:

Do not look back in anger, or forward in fear, but around in awareness.
—James Thurber

Take some time to look around you. What are you aware of?

_____

_____

_____

Today's Focus: _____

Nutritional Intake:

Breakfast _____

Mid-morning_____

Lunch _____

Mid-afternoon _____

Dinner _____

Evening _____

New Foods/Reactions: _____

Stools (amount, number and type): _____

Quick Symptoms Checklist: **Rate Symptoms 0-10**

❏ Headache	❏ Digestive symptoms	Energy level:_____
❏ Joint pain	❏ Abdominal pain	Mood: _____
❏ Muscle pain	❏ Tinnitus	Mental Clarity: _____
❏ Other: _____	❏ Other: _____	Purpose/Hope: _____

My week overall: 0---10

I would describe my week (in one word) as: _____

Because? _____

General progress:

Advanced to a new stage? Y/N   Current stage?_____

New foods tolerated: _____   Foods removed: _____

Animal fats consumed:_____   Avg. daily amount: _____

# of days stock consumed: _____   Avg. daily amount: _____

Probiotics/fermented foods/cultured dairy:

Probiotic supplement: _____Current dose: _____

Die-off symptoms: Y/N   Describe: _____

_____

Beet Kvass _____   Sour Cream _____

Veggie Medley_____   Yogurt _____

Sauerkraut_____   Kefir_____

Detoxing Progress:

# of detox baths: _____ Ingredients: ACV/Epsom/Baking soda

# of days sunbathed: _____ # of minutes per session:_____ minutes

# of days juiced in am: _____in pm: _____

Ingredients:_____

Overall reactions to detoxing: _____

Symptoms descriptions:

Stools: Daily Y/N   #per day _____   Type(s):_____

Digestion: _____

Mood/energy: _____

Memory/clarity: _____

Sleep/Stress: _____

Typical-for-me symptoms: _____

_____

Date _____

❑ FCLO/HVBO	❑ Probiotic	❑ Detox Bath	❑ AM Juicing	❑ Fat
❑ Omega 3/6	❑ Beet Kvass	❑ Oil Pull	❑ PM Juicing	❑ Stock
❑ Iodine	❑ Milk Kefir	❑ Sunbathing	❑ Movement	❑ Ferments

Take a Moment:

"I have done my best." That is about all the philosophy of living one needs. —Lin Yutang

Are you okay with doing your best? Or does that not feel like enough?

_____

_____

_____

Today's Focus: _____

Nutritional Intake:

Breakfast _____

Mid-morning _____

Lunch _____

Mid-afternoon _____

Dinner _____

Evening _____

New Foods/Reactions: _____

Stools (amount, number and type): _____

Quick Symptoms Checklist: **Rate Symptoms 0-10**

❑ Headache	❑ Digestive symptoms	Energy level: _____
❑ Joint pain	❑ Abdominal pain	Mood: _____
❑ Muscle pain	❑ Tinnitus	Mental Clarity: _____
❑ Other: _____	❑ Other: _____	Purpose/Hope: _____

Date _____

❏ FCLO/HVBO	❏ Probiotic	❏ Detox Bath	❏ AM Juicing	❏ Fat
❏ Omega 3/6	❏ Beet Kvass	❏ Oil Pull	❏ PM Juicing	❏ Stock
❏ Iodine	❏ Milk Kefir	❏ Sunbathing	❏ Movement	❏ Ferments

Take a Moment:

Experience is not what happens to a man; it is what a man does with what happens to him. —Aldous Huxley

It is easy to feel like a victim. How else could you approach a bad experience?

_____

_____

_____

Today's Focus: _____

Nutritional Intake:

Breakfast _____

Mid-morning _____

Lunch _____

Mid-afternoon _____

Dinner _____

Evening _____

New Foods/Reactions: _____

Stools (amount, number and type): _____

_____

Quick Symptoms Checklist: Rate Symptoms 0-10

❏ Headache	❏ Digestive symptoms	Energy level:_____
❏ Joint pain	❏ Abdominal pain	Mood: _____
❏ Muscle pain	❏ Tinnitus	Mental Clarity: _____
❏ Other: _____	❏ Other: _____	Purpose/Hope: _____

Date _____

❏ FCLO/HVBO	❏ Probiotic	❏ Detox Bath	❏ AM Juicing	❏ Fat
❏ Omega 3/6	❏ Beet Kvass	❏ Oil Pull	❏ PM Juicing	❏ Stock
❏ Iodine	❏ Milk Kefir	❏ Sunbathing	❏ Movement	❏ Ferments

Take a Moment:

You cannot do a kindness too soon, for you never know
how soon it will be too late. —Ralph Waldo Emerson

What kindness will you do today?

_____

_____

_____

Today's Focus: _____

Nutritional Intake:

Breakfast _____

Mid-morning _____

Lunch _____

Mid-afternoon _____

Dinner _____

Evening _____

New Foods/Reactions: _____

Stools (amount, number and type): _____

_____

Quick Symptoms Checklist: **Rate Symptoms 0-10**

❏ Headache	❏ Digestive symptoms	Energy level:_____
❏ Joint pain	❏ Abdominal pain	Mood: _____
❏ Muscle pain	❏ Tinnitus	Mental Clarity: _____
❏ Other: _____	❏ Other: _____	Purpose/Hope: ____

Date _____

❑ FCLO/HVBO	❑ Probiotic	❑ Detox Bath	❑ AM Juicing	❑ Fat
❑ Omega 3/6	❑ Beet Kvass	❑ Oil Pull	❑ PM Juicing	❑ Stock
❑ Iodine	❑ Milk Kefir	❑ Sunbathing	❑ Movement	❑ Ferments

Take a Moment:

> *Before I get out of bed, I am saying thank you.*
> *I know how important it is to be thankful.* —Al Jarreau

What are you thankful for today?

_____

_____

_____

Today's Focus: _____

Nutritional Intake:

Breakfast _____

Mid-morning_____

Lunch _____

Mid-afternoon _____

Dinner _____

Evening _____

New Foods/Reactions: _____

Stools (amount, number and type): _____

_____

Quick Symptoms Checklist: **Rate Symptoms 0-10**

❑ Headache	❑ Digestive symptoms	Energy level:_____
❑ Joint pain	❑ Abdominal pain	Mood: _____
❑ Muscle pain	❑ Tinnitus	Mental Clarity: _____
❑ Other: _____	❑ Other: _____	Purpose/Hope: _____

Date _____

❏ FCLO/HVBO	❏ Probiotic	❏ Detox Bath	❏ AM Juicing	❏ Fat
❏ Omega 3/6	❏ Beet Kvass	❏ Oil Pull	❏ PM Juicing	❏ Stock
❏ Iodine	❏ Milk Kefir	❏ Sunbathing	❏ Movement	❏ Ferments

Take a Moment:

> *Mistakes are the portals of discovery.* —James Joyce

What have you learned from a recent mistake?

_____

_____

_____

_____

Today's Focus: _____

Nutritional Intake:

Breakfast _____

Mid-morning _____

Lunch _____

Mid-afternoon _____

Dinner _____

Evening _____

New Foods/Reactions: _____

Stools (amount, number and type): _____

_____

Quick Symptoms Checklist: **Rate Symptoms 0-10**

❏ Headache	❏ Digestive symptoms	Energy level:_____
❏ Joint pain	❏ Abdominal pain	Mood: _____
❏ Muscle pain	❏ Tinnitus	Mental Clarity:_____
❏ Other: _____	❏ Other: _____	Purpose/Hope: _____

Date _____

❏ FCLO/HVBO	❏ Probiotic	❏ Detox Bath	❏ AM Juicing	❏ Fat
❏ Omega 3/6	❏ Beet Kvass	❏ Oil Pull	❏ PM Juicing	❏ Stock
❏ Iodine	❏ Milk Kefir	❏ Sunbathing	❏ Movement	❏ Ferments

Take a Moment:

We are all somthing, but none of us are everything. —Blaise Pascal

Do you feel like you have to be everything?

_____

_____

_____

_____

Today's Focus: _____

Nutritional Intake:

Breakfast _____

Mid-morning_____

Lunch _____

Mid-afternoon _____

Dinner _____

Evening _____

New Foods/Reactions: _____

Stools (amount, number and type): _____

_____

Quick Symptoms Checklist: **Rate Symptoms 0-10**

❏ Headache	❏ Digestive symptoms	Energy level:_____
❏ Joint pain	❏ Abdominal pain	Mood: _____
❏ Muscle pain	❏ Tinnitus	Mental Clarity: _____
❏ Other: _____	❏ Other: _____	Purpose/Hope: _____

Date _____

❏ FCLO/HVBO	❏ Probiotic	❏ Detox Bath	❏ AM Juicing	❏ Fat
❏ Omega 3/6	❏ Beet Kvass	❏ Oil Pull	❏ PM Juicing	❏ Stock
❏ Iodine	❏ Milk Kefir	❏ Sunbathing	❏ Movement	❏ Ferments

Take a Moment:

We judge ourselves by what we feel capable of doing, while others judge us by what we have already done. —Henry Wadsworth

How do you judge yourself? Is that how others see you?

_____

_____

_____

Today's Focus: _____

Nutritional Intake:

Breakfast _____

Mid-morning_____

Lunch _____

Mid-afternoon _____

Dinner _____

Evening _____

New Foods/Reactions: _____

Stools (amount, number and type): _____

_____

Quick Symptoms Checklist:		**Rate Symptoms 0-10**
❏ Headache	❏ Digestive symptoms	Energy level:_____
❏ Joint pain	❏ Abdominal pain	Mood: _____
❏ Muscle pain	❏ Tinnitus	Mental Clarity: _____
❏ Other: _____	❏ Other: _____	Purpose/Hope: _____

My week overall: 0--10

I would describe my week (in one word) as: _____

Because? _____

General progress:

Advanced to a new stage? Y/N   Current stage?_____

New foods tolerated: _____   Foods removed: _____

Animal fats consumed: _____   Avg. daily amount: _____

# of days stock consumed: _____   Avg. daily amount: _____

Probiotics/fermented foods/cultured dairy:

Probiotic supplement: _____ Current dose: _____

Die-off symptoms: Y/N   Describe: _____

_____

Beet Kvass _____   Sour Cream _____

Veggie Medley_____   Yogurt _____

Sauerkraut_____   Kefir_____

Detoxing Progress:

# of detox baths: _____ Ingredients: ACV/Epsom/Baking soda

# of days sunbathed: _____ # of minutes per session:_____ minutes

# of days juiced in am: _____in pm: _____

Ingredients:_____

Overall reactions to detoxing: _____

Symptoms descriptions:

Stools: Daily Y/N   #per day _____   Type(s):_____

Digestion: _____

Mood/energy: _____

Memory/clarity: _____

Sleep/Stress: _____

Typical-for-me symptoms: _____

_____

Date _____

❑ FCLO/HVBO	❑ Probiotic	❑ Detox Bath	❑ AM Juicing	❑ Fat
❑ Omega 3/6	❑ Beet Kvass	❑ Oil Pull	❑ PM Juicing	❑ Stock
❑ Iodine	❑ Milk Kefir	❑ Sunbathing	❑ Movement	❑ Ferments

Take a Moment:

> *Life is like an onion; you peel it off one layer at a time*
> *and sometimes you weep.* —Carl Sandburg

Have you experienced this on your health journey?

_____

_____

_____

Today's Focus: _____

Nutritional Intake:

Breakfast _____

Mid-morning_____

Lunch _____

Mid-afternoon _____

Dinner _____

Evening _____

New Foods/Reactions: _____

Stools (amount, number and type): _____

_____

Quick Symptoms Checklist: **Rate Symptoms 0-10**

❑ Headache	❑ Digestive symptoms	Energy level:_____
❑ Joint pain	❑ Abdominal pain	Mood: _____
❑ Muscle pain	❑ Tinnitus	Mental Clarity: _____
❑ Other: _____	❑ Other: _____	Purpose/Hope: _____

Date _____

❏ FCLO/HVBO	❏ Probiotic	❏ Detox Bath	❏ AM Juicing	❏ Fat
❏ Omega 3/6	❏ Beet Kvass	❏ Oil Pull	❏ PM Juicing	❏ Stock
❏ Iodine	❏ Milk Kefir	❏ Sunbathing	❏ Movement	❏ Ferments

Take a Moment:

The best way to cheer yourself up is to try to cheer somebody else up.
—Mark Twain

Who can you cheer up today, and how?

_____

_____

_____

Today's Focus: _____

Nutritional Intake:

Breakfast _____

Mid-morning_____

Lunch _____

Mid-afternoon _____

Dinner _____

Evening _____

New Foods/Reactions: _____

Stools (amount, number and type): _____

Quick Symptoms Checklist: **Rate Symptoms 0-10**

❏ Headache	❏ Digestive symptoms	Energy level:_____
❏ Joint pain	❏ Abdominal pain	Mood: _____
❏ Muscle pain	❏ Tinnitus	Mental Clarity: _____
❏ Other: _____	❏ Other: _____	Purpose/Hope: _____

Date _____

❑ FCLO/HVBO	❑ Probiotic	❑ Detox Bath	❑ AM Juicing	❑ Fat
❑ Omega 3/6	❑ Beet Kvass	❑ Oil Pull	❑ PM Juicing	❑ Stock
❑ Iodine	❑ Milk Kefir	❑ Sunbathing	❑ Movement	❑ Ferments

Take a Moment:

Today or any day that phone may ring and bring good news.
—Ethel Waters

Do you have hope that good is coming?

_____

_____

_____

Today's Focus: _____

Nutritional Intake:

Breakfast _____

Mid-morning_____

Lunch _____

Mid-afternoon _____

Dinner _____

Evening _____

New Foods/Reactions: _____

Stools (amount, number and type): _____

Quick Symptoms Checklist: **Rate Symptoms 0-10**

❑ Headache	❑ Digestive symptoms	Energy level:_____
❑ Joint pain	❑ Abdominal pain	Mood: _____
❑ Muscle pain	❑ Tinnitus	Mental Clarity: _____
❑ Other: _____	❑ Other: _____	Purpose/Hope: _____

Date _____

❏ FCLO/HVBO	❏ Probiotic	❏ Detox Bath	❏ AM Juicing	❏ Fat
❏ Omega 3/6	❏ Beet Kvass	❏ Oil Pull	❏ PM Juicing	❏ Stock
❏ Iodine	❏ Milk Kefir	❏ Sunbathing	❏ Movement	❏ Ferments

Take a Moment:

To succed, you need to find something to hold on to, something to motivate you, something to inspire you. —Tony Dorsett

What is your inspiration or motivation for today?

_____

_____

_____

Today's Focus: _____

Nutritional Intake:

Breakfast _____

Mid-morning_____

Lunch _____

Mid-afternoon _____

Dinner _____

Evening _____

New Foods/Reactions: _____

Stools (amount, number and type): _____

Quick Symptoms Checklist: Rate Symptoms 0-10

❏ Headache	❏ Digestive symptoms	Energy level:_____
❏ Joint pain	❏ Abdominal pain	Mood: _____
❏ Muscle pain	❏ Tinnitus	Mental Clarity: _____
❏ Other: _____	❏ Other: _____	Purpose/Hope: _____

Date _____

❑ FCLO/HVBO	❑ Probiotic	❑ Detox Bath	❑ AM Juicing	❑ Fat
❑ Omega 3/6	❑ Beet Kvass	❑ Oil Pull	❑ PM Juicing	❑ Stock
❑ Iodine	❑ Milk Kefir	❑ Sunbathing	❑ Movement	❑ Ferments

Take a Moment:

Even if you are on the right track, you will get run over if you just sit there. —Will Rogers

We are in a constant state of movement. If we are not taking steps forward, we are losing ground. Do you need to start moving again in something today?

_____

_____

Today's Focus: _____

Nutritional Intake:

Breakfast _____

Mid-morning_____

Lunch _____

Mid-afternoon _____

Dinner _____

Evening _____

New Foods/Reactions: _____

Stools (amount, number and type): _____

Quick Symptoms Checklist: Rate Symptoms 0-10

❑ Headache	❑ Digestive symptoms	Energy level:_____
❑ Joint pain	❑ Abdominal pain	Mood: _____
❑ Muscle pain	❑ Tinnitus	Mental Clarity: _____
❑ Other: _____	❑ Other: _____	Purpose/Hope: _____

Date _____

❑ FCLO/HVBO	❑ Probiotic	❑ Detox Bath	❑ AM Juicing	❑ Fat
❑ Omega 3/6	❑ Beet Kvass	❑ Oil Pull	❑ PM Juicing	❑ Stock
❑ Iodine	❑ Milk Kefir	❑ Sunbathing	❑ Movement	❑ Ferments

Take a Moment:

The absolute truth is the only thing that makes people laugh.
—Carl Reiner

What true story can you tell to make yourself and other people laugh today?

_____

_____

_____

Today's Focus: _____

Nutritional Intake:

Breakfast _____

Mid-morning _____

Lunch _____

Mid-afternoon _____

Dinner _____

Evening _____

New Foods/Reactions: _____

Stools (amount, number and type): _____

Quick Symptoms Checklist:		**Rate Symptoms 0-10**
❑ Headache	❑ Digestive symptoms	Energy level: _____
❑ Joint pain	❑ Abdominal pain	Mood: _____
❑ Muscle pain	❑ Tinnitus	Mental Clarity: _____
❑ Other: _____	❑ Other: _____	Purpose/Hope: _____

Date _____

❑ FCLO/HVBO	❑ Probiotic	❑ Detox Bath	❑ AM Juicing	❑ Fat
❑ Omega 3/6	❑ Beet Kvass	❑ Oil Pull	❑ PM Juicing	❑ Stock
❑ Iodine	❑ Milk Kefir	❑ Sunbathing	❑ Movement	❑ Ferments

Take a Moment:

A good cry lightens the heart. —Yiddish Proverb

Crying is releasing--do you need to release something in tears?

_____

_____

_____

_____

Today's Focus: _____

Nutritional Intake:

Breakfast _____

Mid-morning_____

Lunch _____

Mid-afternoon _____

Dinner _____

Evening _____

New Foods/Reactions:_____

Stools (amount, number and type): _____

_____

Quick Symptoms Checklist:		**Rate Symptoms 0-10**
❑ Headache	❑ Digestive symptoms	Energy level:_____
❑ Joint pain	❑ Abdominal pain	Mood: _____
❑ Muscle pain	❑ Tinnitus	Mental Clarity: _____
❑ Other: _____	❑ Other: _____	Purpose/Hope: _____

My week overall: 0--10

I would describe my week (in one word) as: _____

Because? _____

General progress:

Advanced to a new stage? Y/N   Current stage?_____

New foods tolerated: _____   Foods removed: _____

Animal fats consumed: _____   Avg. daily amount: _____

# of days stock consumed: _____   Avg. daily amount: _____

Probiotics/fermented foods/cultured dairy:

Probiotic supplement: _____Current dose: _____

Die-off symptoms: Y/N   Describe: _____

_____

Beet Kvass _____   Sour Cream _____

Veggie Medley_____   Yogurt _____

Sauerkraut_____   Kefir_____

Detoxing Progress:

# of detox baths: _____ Ingredients: ACV/Epsom/Baking soda

# of days sunbathed: _____ # of minutes per session:_____ minutes

# of days juiced in am: _____in pm: _____

Ingredients:_____

Overall reactions to detoxing: _____

Symptoms descriptions:

Stools: Daily Y/N   #per day _____   Type(s):_____

Digestion: _____

Mood/energy: _____

Memory/clarity: _____

Sleep/Stress: _____

Typical-for-me symptoms: _____

_____

Date _____

❑ FCLO/HVBO	❑ Probiotic	❑ Detox Bath	❑ AM Juicing	❑ Fat
❑ Omega 3/6	❑ Beet Kvass	❑ Oil Pull	❑ PM Juicing	❑ Stock
❑ Iodine	❑ Milk Kefir	❑ Sunbathing	❑ Movement	❑ Ferments

Take a Moment:

In all things of nature there is something of the marvelous. —Aristotle

Take time to admire nature. Describe what you see.

_____

_____

_____

_____

Today's Focus: _____

Nutritional Intake:

Breakfast _____

Mid-morning_____

Lunch _____

Mid-afternoon _____

Dinner _____

Evening _____

New Foods/Reactions: _____

Stools (amount, number and type): _____

_____

Quick Symptoms Checklist:		Rate Symptoms 0-10
❑ Headache	❑ Digestive symptoms	Energy level:_____
❑ Joint pain	❑ Abdominal pain	Mood: _____
❑ Muscle pain	❑ Tinnitus	Mental Clarity: _____
❑ Other: _____	❑ Other: _____	Purpose/Hope: _____

Date _____

❑ FCLO/HVBO	❑ Probiotic	❑ Detox Bath	❑ AM Juicing	❑ Fat
❑ Omega 3/6	❑ Beet Kvass	❑ Oil Pull	❑ PM Juicing	❑ Stock
❑ Iodine	❑ Milk Kefir	❑ Sunbathing	❑ Movement	❑ Ferments

Take a Moment:

> *No great thing is created suddenly.* —Epictetus

Does it feel like this journey is taking forever?

_____

_____

_____

_____

Today's Focus: _____

Nutritional Intake:

Breakfast _____

Mid-morning_____

Lunch _____

Mid-afternoon _____

Dinner _____

Evening _____

New Foods/Reactions: _____

Stools (amount, number and type): _____

Quick Symptoms Checklist: **Rate Symptoms 0-10**

❑ Headache	❑ Digestive symptoms	Energy level:_____
❑ Joint pain	❑ Abdominal pain	Mood: _____
❑ Muscle pain	❑ Tinnitus	Mental Clarity: _____
❑ Other: _____	❑ Other: _____	Purpose/Hope: _____

Date _____

❑ FCLO/HVBO	❑ Probiotic	❑ Detox Bath	❑ AM Juicing	❑ Fat
❑ Omega 3/6	❑ Beet Kvass	❑ Oil Pull	❑ PM Juicing	❑ Stock
❑ Iodine	❑ Milk Kefir	❑ Sunbathing	❑ Movement	❑ Ferments

Take a Moment:

I've always believed that you can think positive just as well as you can think negative. —James A. Baldwin

How are you going to think today?

_____

_____

_____

Today's Focus: _____

Nutritional Intake:

Breakfast _____

Mid-morning_____

Lunch _____

Mid-afternoon _____

Dinner _____

Evening _____

New Foods/Reactions: _____

Stools (amount, number and type): _____

Quick Symptoms Checklist: **Rate Symptoms 0-10**

❑ Headache	❑ Digestive symptoms	Energy level:_____
❑ Joint pain	❑ Abdominal pain	Mood: _____
❑ Muscle pain	❑ Tinnitus	Mental Clarity: _____
❑ Other: _____	❑ Other: _____	Purpose/Hope: _____

Date _____

❏ FCLO/HVBO	❏ Probiotic	❏ Detox Bath	❏ AM Juicing	❏ Fat
❏ Omega 3/6	❏ Beet Kvass	❏ Oil Pull	❏ PM Juicing	❏ Stock
❏ Iodine	❏ Milk Kefir	❏ Sunbathing	❏ Movement	❏ Ferments

Take a Moment:

> *Yesterday is ashes; tomorrow wood.*
> *Only today does the fire burn brightly.* —Eskimo Proverb

How can you live in today?

_____

_____

_____

Today's Focus: _____

Nutritional Intake:

Breakfast _____

Mid-morning_____

Lunch _____

Mid-afternoon _____

Dinner _____

Evening _____

New Foods/Reactions: _____

Stools (amount, number and type): _____

_____

Quick Symptoms Checklist: **Rate Symptoms 0-10**

❏ Headache	❏ Digestive symptoms	Energy level:_____
❏ Joint pain	❏ Abdominal pain	Mood: _____
❏ Muscle pain	❏ Tinnitus	Mental Clarity: _____
❏ Other: _____	❏ Other: _____	Purpose/Hope: _____

Date _____

❑ FCLO/HVBO	❑ Probiotic	❑ Detox Bath	❑ AM Juicing	❑ Fat
❑ Omega 3/6	❑ Beet Kvass	❑ Oil Pull	❑ PM Juicing	❑ Stock
❑ Iodine	❑ Milk Kefir	❑ Sunbathing	❑ Movement	❑ Ferments

Take a Moment:

Your smile will give you a positive countenance that will make people feel comfortable around you. —Les Brown

Do you have a story about something that happened when you smiled?

_____

_____

_____

Today's Focus: _____

Nutritional Intake:

Breakfast _____

Mid-morning _____

Lunch _____

Mid-afternoon _____

Dinner _____

Evening _____

New Foods/Reactions: _____

Stools (amount, number and type): _____

_____

Quick Symptoms Checklist:		Rate Symptoms 0-10
❑ Headache	❑ Digestive symptoms	Energy level:_____
❑ Joint pain	❑ Abdominal pain	Mood: _____
❑ Muscle pain	❑ Tinnitus	Mental Clarity: _____
❑ Other: _____	❑ Other: _____	Purpose/Hope: _____

Date _____

❑ FCLO/HVBO	❑ Probiotic	❑ Detox Bath	❑ AM Juicing	❑ Fat
❑ Omega 3/6	❑ Beet Kvass	❑ Oil Pull	❑ PM Juicing	❑ Stock
❑ Iodine	❑ Milk Kefir	❑ Sunbathing	❑ Movement	❑ Ferments

Take a Moment:

Insanity: doing the same thing over and over again and expecting different results. —Albert Einstein

Are you acting insane in any way? What can you change?

_____

_____

_____

Today's Focus: _____

Nutritional Intake:

Breakfast _____

Mid-morning_____

Lunch _____

Mid-afternoon _____

Dinner _____

Evening _____

New Foods/Reactions: _____

Stools (amount, number and type): _____

_____

Quick Symptoms Checklist:		**Rate Symptoms 0-10**
❑ Headache	❑ Digestive symptoms	Energy level:_____
❑ Joint pain	❑ Abdominal pain	Mood: _____
❑ Muscle pain	❑ Tinnitus	Mental Clarity: _____
❑ Other: _____	❑ Other: _____	Purpose/Hope: _____

Date _____

❏ FCLO/HVBO	❏ Probiotic	❏ Detox Bath	❏ AM Juicing	❏ Fat
❏ Omega 3/6	❏ Beet Kvass	❏ Oil Pull	❏ PM Juicing	❏ Stock
❏ Iodine	❏ Milk Kefir	❏ Sunbathing	❏ Movement	❏ Ferments

Take a Moment:

I've got something inside of me, peasantlike and stubborn, and I'm in it till the end of the race. —Truman Capote

Are you getting tired? What stubborn part can you hold on to that will keep you in until the end?

_____

_____

_____

Today's Focus: _____

Nutritional Intake:

Breakfast _____

Mid-morning_____

Lunch _____

Mid-afternoon _____

Dinner _____

Evening _____

New Foods/Reactions:_____

Stools (amount, number and type): _____

_____

Quick Symptoms Checklist: **Rate Symptoms 0-10**

❏ Headache	❏ Digestive symptoms	Energy level:_____
❏ Joint pain	❏ Abdominal pain	Mood: _____
❏ Muscle pain	❏ Tinnitus	Mental Clarity:_____
❏ Other: _____	❏ Other: _____	Purpose/Hope:_____

My week overall: 0--**10**

I would describe my week (in one word) as: _____

Because? _____

General progress:

Advanced to a new stage? Y/N   Current stage?_____

New foods tolerated: _____   Foods removed: _____

Animal fats consumed:_____   Avg. daily amount: _____

# of days stock consumed: _____   Avg. daily amount: _____

Probiotics/fermented foods/cultured dairy:

Probiotic supplement: _____Current dose: _____

Die-off symptoms: Y/N   Describe: _____

_____

Beet Kvass_____   Sour Cream_____

Veggie Medley_____   Yogurt _____

Sauerkraut_____   Kefir_____

Detoxing Progress:

# of detox baths: _____ Ingredients: ACV/Epsom/Baking soda

# of days sunbathed: _____ # of minutes per session:_____ minutes

# of days juiced in am: _____in pm: _____

Ingredients:_____

Overall reactions to detoxing: _____

Symptoms descriptions:

Stools: Daily Y/N   #per day _____   Type(s):_____

Digestion: _____

Mood/energy: _____

Memory/clarity: _____

Sleep/Stress: _____

Typical-for-me symptoms: _____

_____

Date _____

❑ FCLO/HVBO	❑ Probiotic	❑ Detox Bath	❑ AM Juicing	❑ Fat
❑ Omega 3/6	❑ Beet Kvass	❑ Oil Pull	❑ PM Juicing	❑ Stock
❑ Iodine	❑ Milk Kefir	❑ Sunbathing	❑ Movement	❑ Ferments

Take a Moment:

> *The best way out is always through.* —Robert Frost

What will help you get through?

_____

_____

_____

_____

Today's Focus: _____

Nutritional Intake:

Breakfast _____

Mid-morning_____

Lunch _____

Mid-afternoon _____

Dinner _____

Evening _____

New Foods/Reactions: _____

Stools (amount, number and type): _____

Quick Symptoms Checklist: **Rate Symptoms 0-10**

❑ Headache	❑ Digestive symptoms	Energy level:_____
❑ Joint pain	❑ Abdominal pain	Mood: _____
❑ Muscle pain	❑ Tinnitus	Mental Clarity: _____
❑ Other: _____	❑ Other: _____	Purpose/Hope: _____

Date _____

❏ FCLO/HVBO	❏ Probiotic	❏ Detox Bath	❏ AM Juicing	❏ Fat
❏ Omega 3/6	❏ Beet Kvass	❏ Oil Pull	❏ PM Juicing	❏ Stock
❏ Iodine	❏ Milk Kefir	❏ Sunbathing	❏ Movement	❏ Ferments

Take a Moment:

That which we obtain too easily, we esteem too lightly. —Thomas Paine

You are working hard for something right now. Reflect on the value you are creating!

_____

_____

_____

Today's Focus: _____

Nutritional Intake:

Breakfast _____

Mid-morning _____

Lunch _____

Mid-afternoon _____

Dinner _____

Evening _____

New Foods/Reactions: _____

Stools (amount, number and type): _____

_____

Quick Symptoms Checklist: **Rate Symptoms 0-10**

❏ Headache	❏ Digestive symptoms	Energy level:_____
❏ Joint pain	❏ Abdominal pain	Mood: _____
❏ Muscle pain	❏ Tinnitus	Mental Clarity:_____
❏ Other: _____	❏ Other: _____	Purpose/Hope: _____

Date _____

❑ FCLO/HVBO	❑ Probiotic	❑ Detox Bath	❑ AM Juicing	❑ Fat
❑ Omega 3/6	❑ Beet Kvass	❑ Oil Pull	❑ PM Juicing	❑ Stock
❑ Iodine	❑ Milk Kefir	❑ Sunbathing	❑ Movement	❑ Ferments

Take a Moment:

To be wronged is nothing unless you continue to remember it.
—Confucius

This can be hard to practice. Is there something that you are remembering that is weighing you down?

_____

_____

Today's Focus: _____

Nutritional Intake:

Breakfast _____

Mid-morning_____

Lunch _____

Mid-afternoon _____

Dinner _____

Evening _____

New Foods/Reactions: _____

Stools (amount, number and type): _____

Quick Symptoms Checklist: **Rate Symptoms 0-10**

❑ Headache	❑ Digestive symptoms	Energy level:_____
❑ Joint pain	❑ Abdominal pain	Mood: _____
❑ Muscle pain	❑ Tinnitus	Mental Clarity: _____
❑ Other: _____	❑ Other: _____	Purpose/Hope: _____

Date _____

❑ FCLO/HVBO	❑ Probiotic	❑ Detox Bath	❑ AM Juicing	❑ Fat
❑ Omega 3/6	❑ Beet Kvass	❑ Oil Pull	❑ PM Juicing	❑ Stock
❑ Iodine	❑ Milk Kefir	❑ Sunbathing	❑ Movement	❑ Ferments

Take a Moment:

Grant that we may not so much seek to be consoled as to console.
To be understood as to understand. —St. Francis of Assisi

We all want to be better understood. Who can you work to understand better today?

_____

_____

Today's Focus: _____

Nutritional Intake:

Breakfast _____

Mid-morning_____

Lunch _____

Mid-afternoon _____

Dinner _____

Evening _____

New Foods/Reactions: _____

Stools (amount, number and type): _____

_____

Quick Symptoms Checklist: Rate Symptoms 0-10

❑ Headache	❑ Digestive symptoms	Energy level:_____
❑ Joint pain	❑ Abdominal pain	Mood: _____
❑ Muscle pain	❑ Tinnitus	Mental Clarity: _____
❑ Other: _____	❑ Other: _____	Purpose/Hope: _____

Date _____

❑ FCLO/HVBO	❑ Probiotic	❑ Detox Bath	❑ AM Juicing	❑ Fat
❑ Omega 3/6	❑ Beet Kvass	❑ Oil Pull	❑ PM Juicing	❑ Stock
❑ Iodine	❑ Milk Kefir	❑ Sunbathing	❑ Movement	❑ Ferments

Take a Moment:

Well begun is half done. —Aristotle

What can you begin well today?

_____

_____

_____

_____

Today's Focus: _____

Nutritional Intake:

Breakfast _____

Mid-morning_____

Lunch _____

Mid-afternoon _____

Dinner _____

Evening _____

New Foods/Reactions: _____

Stools (amount, number and type): _____

_____

Quick Symptoms Checklist: **Rate Symptoms 0-10**

❑ Headache	❑ Digestive symptoms	Energy level:_____
❑ Joint pain	❑ Abdominal pain	Mood: _____
❑ Muscle pain	❑ Tinnitus	Mental Clarity: _____
❑ Other: _____	❑ Other: _____	Purpose/Hope: _____

Date _____

❑ FCLO/HVBO	❑ Probiotic	❑ Detox Bath	❑ AM Juicing	❑ Fat
❑ Omega 3/6	❑ Beet Kvass	❑ Oil Pull	❑ PM Juicing	❑ Stock
❑ Iodine	❑ Milk Kefir	❑ Sunbathing	❑ Movement	❑ Ferments

Take a Moment:

We must not, in trying to think about how we can make a big difference, ignore the small daily differences we can make which, over time, add up to big differences that we often cannot foresee. —Marian Wright Edelman

Have you given up making small daily differences? Which ones do you want to start making again?

_____

_____

Today's Focus: _____

Nutritional Intake:

Breakfast _____

Mid-morning_____

Lunch _____

Mid-afternoon _____

Dinner _____

Evening _____

New Foods/Reactions: _____

Stools (amount, number and type): _____

_____

Quick Symptoms Checklist: **Rate Symptoms 0-10**

❑ Headache	❑ Digestive symptoms	Energy level:_____
❑ Joint pain	❑ Abdominal pain	Mood: _____
❑ Muscle pain	❑ Tinnitus	Mental Clarity:_____
❑ Other: _____	❑ Other: _____	Purpose/Hope: _____

Date _____

❏ FCLO/HVBO	❏ Probiotic	❏ Detox Bath	❏ AM Juicing	❏ Fat
❏ Omega 3/6	❏ Beet Kvass	❏ Oil Pull	❏ PM Juicing	❏ Stock
❏ Iodine	❏ Milk Kefir	❏ Sunbathing	❏ Movement	❏ Ferments

Take a Moment:

Look deep into nature, and then you will understand everything better.
—Albert Einstein

Take time to be in a nature today. Write about your thoughts.

_____

_____

_____

Today's Focus: _____

Nutritional Intake:

Breakfast _____

Mid-morning_____

Lunch _____

Mid-afternoon _____

Dinner _____

Evening _____

New Foods/Reactions: _____

Stools (amount, number and type): _____

Quick Symptoms Checklist: **Rate Symptoms 0-10**

❏ Headache	❏ Digestive symptoms	Energy level:_____
❏ Joint pain	❏ Abdominal pain	Mood: _____
❏ Muscle pain	❏ Tinnitus	Mental Clarity: _____
❏ Other: _____	❏ Other: _____	Purpose/Hope: _____

My week overall: 0---10

I would describe my week (in one word) as: _____

Because? _____

General progress:

Advanced to a new stage? Y/N   Current stage?_____

New foods tolerated: _____   Foods removed: _____

Animal fats consumed: _____   Avg. daily amount: _____

# of days stock consumed: _____   Avg. daily amount: _____

Probiotics/fermented foods/cultured dairy:

Probiotic supplement: _____ Current dose: _____

Die-off symptoms: Y/N   Describe: _____

_____

Beet Kvass _____   Sour Cream _____

Veggie Medley _____   Yogurt _____

Sauerkraut _____   Kefir _____

Detoxing Progress:

# of detox baths: _____   Ingredients: ACV/Epsom/Baking soda

# of days sunbathed: _____   # of minutes per session: _____ minutes

# of days juiced in am: _____ in pm: _____

Ingredients: _____

Overall reactions to detoxing: _____

Symptoms descriptions:

Stools: Daily Y/N   #per day _____   Type(s): _____

Digestion: _____

Mood/energy: _____

Memory/clarity: _____

Sleep/Stress: _____

Typical-for-me symptoms: _____

_____

Date _____

❏ FCLO/HVBO	❏ Probiotic	❏ Detox Bath	❏ AM Juicing	❏ Fat
❏ Omega 3/6	❏ Beet Kvass	❏ Oil Pull	❏ PM Juicing	❏ Stock
❏ Iodine	❏ Milk Kefir	❏ Sunbathing	❏ Movement	❏ Ferments

Take a Moment:

If you can't feed a hundred people, then just feed one. —Mother Teresa

It's easy to feel overwhelmed at all that you could do.
Don't be paralyzed. What can you do?

_____

_____

_____

Today's Focus: _____

Nutritional Intake:

Breakfast _____

Mid-morning_____

Lunch _____

Mid-afternoon _____

Dinner _____

Evening _____

New Foods/Reactions: _____

Stools (amount, number and type): _____

Quick Symptoms Checklist: **Rate Symptoms 0-10**

❏ Headache	❏ Digestive symptoms	Energy level:_____
❏ Joint pain	❏ Abdominal pain	Mood: _____
❏ Muscle pain	❏ Tinnitus	Mental Clarity: _____
❏ Other: _____	❏ Other: _____	Purpose/Hope: _____

Date _____

☐ FCLO/HVBO ☐ Probiotic ☐ Detox Bath ☐ AM Juicing ☐ Fat
☐ Omega 3/6 ☐ Beet Kvass ☐ Oil Pull ☐ PM Juicing ☐ Stock
☐ Iodine ☐ Milk Kefir ☐ Sunbathing ☐ Movement ☐ Ferments

Take a Moment:

Be happy for this moment. This moment is your life. —Omar Khayyam

Are you happy in this moment? Why or why not?

_____

_____

_____

_____

Today's Focus: _____

Nutritional Intake:

Breakfast _____

Mid-morning _____

Lunch _____

Mid-afternoon _____

Dinner _____

Evening _____

New Foods/Reactions: _____

Stools (amount, number and type): _____

_____

Quick Symptoms Checklist: **Rate Symptoms 0-10**

☐ Headache   ☐ Digestive symptoms   Energy level: _____
☐ Joint pain   ☐ Abdominal pain   Mood: _____
☐ Muscle pain   ☐ Tinnitus   Mental Clarity: _____
☐ Other: _____   ☐ Other: _____   Purpose/Hope: _____

Date _____

❑ FCLO/HVBO	❑ Probiotic	❑ Detox Bath	❑ AM Juicing	❑ Fat
❑ Omega 3/6	❑ Beet Kvass	❑ Oil Pull	❑ PM Juicing	❑ Stock
❑ Iodine	❑ Milk Kefir	❑ Sunbathing	❑ Movement	❑ Ferments

Take a Moment:

>   *Teach us delight in simple things.* —Rudyard Kippling

Don't push aside simple delights. What small things make you smile?

_____

_____

_____

_____

Today's Focus: _____

Nutritional Intake:

Breakfast _____

Mid-morning_____

Lunch _____

Mid-afternoon _____

Dinner _____

Evening _____

New Foods/Reactions:_____

Stools (amount, number and type): _____

_____

Quick Symptoms Checklist: **Rate Symptoms 0-10**

❑ Headache	❑ Digestive symptoms	Energy level:_____
❑ Joint pain	❑ Abdominal pain	Mood: _____
❑ Muscle pain	❑ Tinnitus	Mental Clarity: _____
❑ Other: _____	❑ Other: _____	Purpose/Hope: _____

Date _____

❏ FCLO/HVBO	❏ Probiotic	❏ Detox Bath	❏ AM Juicing	❏ Fat
❏ Omega 3/6	❏ Beet Kvass	❏ Oil Pull	❏ PM Juicing	❏ Stock
❏ Iodine	❏ Milk Kefir	❏ Sunbathing	❏ Movement	❏ Ferments

Take a Moment:

It is not by spectacular achievements that man can be transformed, but by will. —Henrik Ibsen

How do you keep going?

_____

_____

_____

Today's Focus: _____

Nutritional Intake:

Breakfast _____

Mid-morning_____

Lunch _____

Mid-afternoon _____

Dinner _____

Evening _____

New Foods/Reactions: _____

Stools (amount, number and type): _____

_____

Quick Symptoms Checklist: **Rate Symptoms 0-10**

❏ Headache	❏ Digestive symptoms	Energy level:_____
❏ Joint pain	❏ Abdominal pain	Mood: _____
❏ Muscle pain	❏ Tinnitus	Mental Clarity:_____
❏ Other: _____	❏ Other: _____	Purpose/Hope: _____

Date _____

❏ FCLO/HVBO	❏ Probiotic	❏ Detox Bath	❏ AM Juicing	❏ Fat
❏ Omega 3/6	❏ Beet Kvass	❏ Oil Pull	❏ PM Juicing	❏ Stock
❏ Iodine	❏ Milk Kefir	❏ Sunbathing	❏ Movement	❏ Ferments

Take a Moment:

Health and cheerfulness naturally beget each other. —Joseph Addison

What are you cheerful about today?

_____

_____

_____

_____

Today's Focus: _____

Nutritional Intake:

Breakfast _____

Mid-morning _____

Lunch _____

Mid-afternoon _____

Dinner _____

Evening _____

New Foods/Reactions: _____

Stools (amount, number and type): _____

_____

Quick Symptoms Checklist: **Rate Symptoms 0-10**

❏ Headache	❏ Digestive symptoms	Energy level:_____
❏ Joint pain	❏ Abdominal pain	Mood: _____
❏ Muscle pain	❏ Tinnitus	Mental Clarity: _____
❏ Other: _____	❏ Other: _____	Purpose/Hope: _____

Date _____

❏ FCLO/HVBO	❏ Probiotic	❏ Detox Bath	❏ AM Juicing	❏ Fat
❏ Omega 3/6	❏ Beet Kvass	❏ Oil Pull	❏ PM Juicing	❏ Stock
❏ Iodine	❏ Milk Kefir	❏ Sunbathing	❏ Movement	❏ Ferments

Take a Moment:

Humor is our way of defending ourselves from life's absurdities by thinking absurdly about them. —Lewis Mumford

Write about the humor in a recent hard life moment.

_____

_____

_____

Today's Focus: _____

Nutritional Intake:

Breakfast _____

Mid-morning _____

Lunch _____

Mid-afternoon _____

Dinner _____

Evening _____

New Foods/Reactions: _____

Stools (amount, number and type): _____

_____

Quick Symptoms Checklist: Rate Symptoms 0-10

❏ Headache	❏ Digestive symptoms	Energy level:_____
❏ Joint pain	❏ Abdominal pain	Mood: _____
❏ Muscle pain	❏ Tinnitus	Mental Clarity:_____
❏ Other: _____	❏ Other: _____	Purpose/Hope: _____

Date _____

❏ FCLO/HVBO	❏ Probiotic	❏ Detox Bath	❏ AM Juicing	❏ Fat
❏ Omega 3/6	❏ Beet Kvass	❏ Oil Pull	❏ PM Juicing	❏ Stock
❏ Iodine	❏ Milk Kefir	❏ Sunbathing	❏ Movement	❏ Ferments

Take a Moment:

Sometimes life hits you in the head with a brick. Don't loose faith.
—Steve Jobs

Have you been hit with a brick. Take some time to grieve today.

_____

_____

_____

Today's Focus: _____

Nutritional Intake:

Breakfast _____

Mid-morning_____

Lunch _____

Mid-afternoon _____

Dinner _____

Evening _____

New Foods/Reactions:_____

Stools (amount, number and type): _____

Quick Symptoms Checklist: **Rate Symptoms 0-10**

❏ Headache	❏ Digestive symptoms	Energy level:_____
❏ Joint pain	❏ Abdominal pain	Mood: _____
❏ Muscle pain	❏ Tinnitus	Mental Clarity: _____
❏ Other: _____	❏ Other: _____	Purpose/Hope: _____

My week overall: 0---10

I would describe my week (in one word) as: _____

Because? _____

General progress:

Advanced to a new stage? Y/N   Current stage?_____

New foods tolerated: _____   Foods removed: _____

Animal fats consumed:_____   Avg. daily amount: _____

# of days stock consumed: _____   Avg. daily amount: _____

Probiotics/fermented foods/cultured dairy:

Probiotic supplement: _____Current dose: _____

Die-off symptoms: Y/N   Describe: _____

_____

Beet Kvass _____   Sour Cream_____

Veggie Medley_____   Yogurt _____

Sauerkraut_____   Kefir_____

Detoxing Progress:

# of detox baths: _____ Ingredients: ACV/Epsom/Baking soda

# of days sunbathed: _____ # of minutes per session:_____ minutes

# of days juiced in am: _____in pm: _____

Ingredients:_____

Overall reactions to detoxing: _____

Symptoms descriptions:

Stools: Daily Y/N   #per day _____   Type(s):_____

Digestion: _____

Mood/energy: _____

Memory/clarity: _____

Sleep/Stress: _____

Typical-for-me symptoms: _____

_____

Date _____

❑ FCLO/HVBO	❑ Probiotic	❑ Detox Bath	❑ AM Juicing	❑ Fat
❑ Omega 3/6	❑ Beet Kvass	❑ Oil Pull	❑ PM Juicing	❑ Stock
❑ Iodine	❑ Milk Kefir	❑ Sunbathing	❑ Movement	❑ Ferments

Take a Moment:

> *We are made to persist. That's how we find out who we are.*
> —Tobias Wolff

As you persist in life, who are you finding yourself to be?

_____

_____

_____

Today's Focus: _____

Nutritional Intake:

Breakfast _____

Mid-morning _____

Lunch _____

Mid-afternoon _____

Dinner _____

Evening _____

New Foods/Reactions: _____

Stools (amount, number and type): _____

_____

Quick Symptoms Checklist: **Rate Symptoms 0-10**

❑ Headache	❑ Digestive symptoms	Energy level:_____
❑ Joint pain	❑ Abdominal pain	Mood: _____
❑ Muscle pain	❑ Tinnitus	Mental Clarity: _____
❑ Other: _____	❑ Other: _____	Purpose/Hope: _____

Date _____

❏ FCLO/HVBO	❏ Probiotic	❏ Detox Bath	❏ AM Juicing	❏ Fat
❏ Omega 3/6	❏ Beet Kvass	❏ Oil Pull	❏ PM Juicing	❏ Stock
❏ Iodine	❏ Milk Kefir	❏ Sunbathing	❏ Movement	❏ Ferments

Take a Moment:

Pick battles big enough to matter, small enough to win.
—Jonathan Kozol

We face many battles. What battle are you going to pick today?

_____

_____

_____

Today's Focus: _____

Nutritional Intake:

Breakfast _____

Mid-morning _____

Lunch _____

Mid-afternoon _____

Dinner _____

Evening _____

New Foods/Reactions: _____

Stools (amount, number and type): _____

_____

Quick Symptoms Checklist: **Rate Symptoms 0-10**

❏ Headache	❏ Digestive symptoms	Energy level:_____
❏ Joint pain	❏ Abdominal pain	Mood: _____
❏ Muscle pain	❏ Tinnitus	Mental Clarity:_____
❏ Other: _____	❏ Other: _____	Purpose/Hope: _____

Date _____

❏ FCLO/HVBO	❏ Probiotic	❏ Detox Bath	❏ AM Juicing	❏ Fat
❏ Omega 3/6	❏ Beet Kvass	❏ Oil Pull	❏ PM Juicing	❏ Stock
❏ Iodine	❏ Milk Kefir	❏ Sunbathing	❏ Movement	❏ Ferments

Take a Moment:

Life is an adventure in forgiveness. —Norman Cousins

Grudges and anger can be as toxic as heavy metals in our body. Is there someone you should forgive today?

_____

_____

_____

Today's Focus: _____

Nutritional Intake:

Breakfast _____

Mid-morning_____

Lunch _____

Mid-afternoon _____

Dinner _____

Evening _____

New Foods/Reactions: _____

Stools (amount, number and type): _____

_____

Quick Symptoms Checklist: Rate Symptoms 0-10

❏ Headache	❏ Digestive symptoms	Energy level:_____
❏ Joint pain	❏ Abdominal pain	Mood: _____
❏ Muscle pain	❏ Tinnitus	Mental Clarity: _____
❏ Other: _____	❏ Other: _____	Purpose/Hope: _____

Date _____

❑ FCLO/HVBO	❑ Probiotic	❑ Detox Bath	❑ AM Juicing	❑ Fat
❑ Omega 3/6	❑ Beet Kvass	❑ Oil Pull	❑ PM Juicing	❑ Stock
❑ Iodine	❑ Milk Kefir	❑ Sunbathing	❑ Movement	❑ Ferments

Take a Moment:

> *Beware the barrenness of a busy life.* —Socrates

Are you busy? Has it made your life barren? In what way?

_____

_____

_____

_____

Today's Focus: _____

Nutritional Intake:

Breakfast _____

Mid-morning _____

Lunch _____

Mid-afternoon _____

Dinner _____

Evening _____

New Foods/Reactions: _____

Stools (amount, number and type): _____

Quick Symptoms Checklist:		Rate Symptoms 0-10
❑ Headache	❑ Digestive symptoms	Energy level: _____
❑ Joint pain	❑ Abdominal pain	Mood: _____
❑ Muscle pain	❑ Tinnitus	Mental Clarity: _____
❑ Other: _____	❑ Other: _____	Purpose/Hope: _____

Date _____

❏ FCLO/HVBO	❏ Probiotic	❏ Detox Bath	❏ AM Juicing	❏ Fat
❏ Omega 3/6	❏ Beet Kvass	❏ Oil Pull	❏ PM Juicing	❏ Stock
❏ Iodine	❏ Milk Kefir	❏ Sunbathing	❏ Movement	❏ Ferments

Take a Moment:

Always do your best. What you plant now, you will harvest later.
—Og Mandino

What do you want to harvest later?

_____

_____

_____

Today's Focus: _____

Nutritional Intake:

Breakfast _____

Mid-morning _____

Lunch _____

Mid-afternoon _____

Dinner _____

Evening _____

New Foods/Reactions: _____

Stools (amount, number and type): _____

Quick Symptoms Checklist: **Rate Symptoms 0-10**

❏ Headache	❏ Digestive symptoms	Energy level:_____
❏ Joint pain	❏ Abdominal pain	Mood: _____
❏ Muscle pain	❏ Tinnitus	Mental Clarity: _____
❏ Other: _____	❏ Other: _____	Purpose/Hope: _____

Date _____

❏ FCLO/HVBO	❏ Probiotic	❏ Detox Bath	❏ AM Juicing	❏ Fat
❏ Omega 3/6	❏ Beet Kvass	❏ Oil Pull	❏ PM Juicing	❏ Stock
❏ Iodine	❏ Milk Kefir	❏ Sunbathing	❏ Movement	❏ Ferments

Take a Moment:

A strong positive mental attitude will create more miracles than any wonder drug. —Patricia Neal

What helps you keep a positive mental attitude?

_____

_____

_____

Today's Focus: _____

Nutritional Intake:

Breakfast _____

Mid-morning _____

Lunch _____

Mid-afternoon _____

Dinner _____

Evening _____

New Foods/Reactions: _____

Stools (amount, number and type): _____

_____

Quick Symptoms Checklist: **Rate Symptoms 0-10**

❏ Headache	❏ Digestive symptoms	Energy level:_____
❏ Joint pain	❏ Abdominal pain	Mood: _____
❏ Muscle pain	❏ Tinnitus	Mental Clarity:_____
❏ Other: _____	❏ Other: _____	Purpose/Hope: _____

Date _____

❏ FCLO/HVBO	❏ Probiotic	❏ Detox Bath	❏ AM Juicing	❏ Fat
❏ Omega 3/6	❏ Beet Kvass	❏ Oil Pull	❏ PM Juicing	❏ Stock
❏ Iodine	❏ Milk Kefir	❏ Sunbathing	❏ Movement	❏ Ferments

Take a Moment:

Opportunity is missed by most people because it is dressed in overalls and looks like work. —Thomas Edison

Think for a minute—are you missing an opportunity to get something you want because it looks like work?

_____

_____

_____

Today's Focus: _____

Nutritional Intake:

Breakfast _____

Mid-morning _____

Lunch _____

Mid-afternoon _____

Dinner _____

Evening _____

New Foods/Reactions: _____

Stools (amount, number and type): _____

Quick Symptoms Checklist: **Rate Symptoms 0-10**

❏ Headache	❏ Digestive symptoms	Energy level:_____
❏ Joint pain	❏ Abdominal pain	Mood: _____
❏ Muscle pain	❏ Tinnitus	Mental Clarity: _____
❏ Other: _____	❏ Other: _____	Purpose/Hope: _____

My week overall: 0--**10**

I would describe my week (in one word) as: _____

Because? _____

General progress:

Advanced to a new stage? Y/N   Current stage?_____

New foods tolerated: _____   Foods removed: _____

Animal fats consumed: _____   Avg. daily amount: _____

# of days stock consumed: _____   Avg. daily amount: _____

Probiotics/fermented foods/cultured dairy:

Probiotic supplement: _____Current dose: _____

Die-off symptoms: Y/N   Describe: _____

_____

Beet Kvass_____   Sour Cream_____

Veggie Medley_____   Yogurt _____

Sauerkraut_____   Kefir_____

Detoxing Progress:

# of detox baths: _____ Ingredients: ACV/Epsom/Baking soda

# of days sunbathed: _____ # of minutes per session:_____ minutes

# of days juiced in am: _____in pm: _____

Ingredients:_____

Overall reactions to detoxing: _____

Symptoms descriptions:

Stools: Daily Y/N   #per day _____   Type(s):_____

Digestion: _____

Mood/energy: _____

Memory/clarity: _____

Sleep/Stress: _____

Typical-for-me symptoms: _____

_____

Date _____

❑ FCLO/HVBO	❑ Probiotic	❑ Detox Bath	❑ AM Juicing	❑ Fat
❑ Omega 3/6	❑ Beet Kvass	❑ Oil Pull	❑ PM Juicing	❑ Stock
❑ Iodine	❑ Milk Kefir	❑ Sunbathing	❑ Movement	❑ Ferments

Take a Moment:

When nothing is sure, everything is possible. —Margaret Drabble

It takes a lot of courage to believe this—what do you think about it?

_____

_____

_____

_____

Today's Focus: _____

Nutritional Intake:

Breakfast _____

Mid-morning _____

Lunch _____

Mid-afternoon _____

Dinner _____

Evening _____

New Foods/Reactions: _____

Stools (amount, number and type): _____

Quick Symptoms Checklist: **Rate Symptoms 0-10**

❑ Headache	❑ Digestive symptoms	Energy level: _____
❑ Joint pain	❑ Abdominal pain	Mood: _____
❑ Muscle pain	❑ Tinnitus	Mental Clarity: _____
❑ Other: _____	❑ Other: _____	Purpose/Hope: ____

Date _____

❏ FCLO/HVBO	❏ Probiotic	❏ Detox Bath	❏ AM Juicing	❏ Fat
❏ Omega 3/6	❏ Beet Kvass	❏ Oil Pull	❏ PM Juicing	❏ Stock
❏ Iodine	❏ Milk Kefir	❏ Sunbathing	❏ Movement	❏ Ferments

Take a Moment:

You express the truth of your character with the choice of your actions.
—Steve Maraboli

What do you choose to do today?

_____

_____

_____

Today's Focus: _____

Nutritional Intake:

Breakfast _____

Mid-morning_____

Lunch _____

Mid-afternoon _____

Dinner _____

Evening _____

New Foods/Reactions: _____

Stools (amount, number and type): _____

_____

Quick Symptoms Checklist: Rate Symptoms 0-10

❏ Headache	❏ Digestive symptoms	Energy level:_____
❏ Joint pain	❏ Abdominal pain	Mood: _____
❏ Muscle pain	❏ Tinnitus	Mental Clarity: _____
❏ Other: _____	❏ Other: _____	Purpose/Hope: _____

Date _____

❏ FCLO/HVBO	❏ Probiotic	❏ Detox Bath	❏ AM Juicing	❏ Fat
❏ Omega 3/6	❏ Beet Kvass	❏ Oil Pull	❏ PM Juicing	❏ Stock
❏ Iodine	❏ Milk Kefir	❏ Sunbathing	❏ Movement	❏ Ferments

Take a Moment:

Laugh my friend, for laughter ignites a fire within the pit of your belly and awakens your being. —Stella McCartney

What made you laugh today?

_____

_____

_____

Today's Focus: _____

Nutritional Intake:

Breakfast _____

Mid-morning_____

Lunch _____

Mid-afternoon _____

Dinner _____

Evening _____

New Foods/Reactions:_____

Stools (amount, number and type): _____

Quick Symptoms Checklist: **Rate Symptoms 0-10**

❏ Headache	❏ Digestive symptoms	Energy level:_____
❏ Joint pain	❏ Abdominal pain	Mood: _____
❏ Muscle pain	❏ Tinnitus	Mental Clarity:_____
❏ Other: _____	❏ Other: _____	Purpose/Hope: _____

Date _____

❏ FCLO/HVBO	❏ Probiotic	❏ Detox Bath	❏ AM Juicing	❏ Fat
❏ Omega 3/6	❏ Beet Kvass	❏ Oil Pull	❏ PM Juicing	❏ Stock
❏ Iodine	❏ Milk Kefir	❏ Sunbathing	❏ Movement	❏ Ferments

Take a Moment:

No act of kindness, no matter how small, is ever wasted. —Aesop

What act of kindness will you do today?

_____

_____

_____

_____

Today's Focus: _____

Nutritional Intake:

Breakfast _____

Mid-morning _____

Lunch _____

Mid-afternoon _____

Dinner _____

Evening _____

New Foods/Reactions: _____

Stools (amount, number and type): _____

Quick Symptoms Checklist: **Rate Symptoms 0-10**

❏ Headache	❏ Digestive symptoms	Energy level: _____
❏ Joint pain	❏ Abdominal pain	Mood: _____
❏ Muscle pain	❏ Tinnitus	Mental Clarity: _____
❏ Other: _____	❏ Other: _____	Purpose/Hope: _____

Date _____

❑ FCLO/HVBO	❑ Probiotic	❑ Detox Bath	❑ AM Juicing	❑ Fat
❑ Omega 3/6	❑ Beet Kvass	❑ Oil Pull	❑ PM Juicing	❑ Stock
❑ Iodine	❑ Milk Kefir	❑ Sunbathing	❑ Movement	❑ Ferments

Take a Moment:

I am grateful for what I have. My thanksgiving is perpetual.
—Henry David Thoreau

What are you grateful for today?

_____

_____

_____

Today's Focus: _____

Nutritional Intake:

Breakfast _____

Mid-morning_____

Lunch _____

Mid-afternoon _____

Dinner _____

Evening _____

New Foods/Reactions: _____

Stools (amount, number and type): _____

Quick Symptoms Checklist: **Rate Symptoms 0-10**

❑ Headache	❑ Digestive symptoms	Energy level:_____
❑ Joint pain	❑ Abdominal pain	Mood: _____
❑ Muscle pain	❑ Tinnitus	Mental Clarity: _____
❑ Other: _____	❑ Other: _____	Purpose/Hope: _____

Date _____

❏ FCLO/HVBO	❏ Probiotic	❏ Detox Bath	❏ AM Juicing	❏ Fat
❏ Omega 3/6	❏ Beet Kvass	❏ Oil Pull	❏ PM Juicing	❏ Stock
❏ Iodine	❏ Milk Kefir	❏ Sunbathing	❏ Movement	❏ Ferments

Take a Moment:

*If you're not making mistakes, then you're not doing anything.
I'm positive that a doer makes mistakes.* —John Wooden

Are you doing things? The proof is in your mistakes.

_____

_____

_____

Today's Focus: _____

Nutritional Intake:

Breakfast _____

Mid-morning_____

Lunch _____

Mid-afternoon _____

Dinner _____

Evening _____

New Foods/Reactions: _____

Stools (amount, number and type): _____

_____

Quick Symptoms Checklist: **Rate Symptoms 0-10**

❏ Headache	❏ Digestive symptoms	Energy level:_____
❏ Joint pain	❏ Abdominal pain	Mood: _____
❏ Muscle pain	❏ Tinnitus	Mental Clarity:_____
❏ Other: _____	❏ Other: _____	Purpose/Hope: _____

Date _____

❑ FCLO/HVBO	❑ Probiotic	❑ Detox Bath	❑ AM Juicing	❑ Fat
❑ Omega 3/6	❑ Beet Kvass	❑ Oil Pull	❑ PM Juicing	❑ Stock
❑ Iodine	❑ Milk Kefir	❑ Sunbathing	❑ Movement	❑ Ferments

Take a Moment:

Life is really simple, but we insist on making it complicated.
—Confucius

How can you uncomplicate your life today?

_____

_____

_____

Today's Focus: _____

Nutritional Intake:

Breakfast _____

Mid-morning_____

Lunch _____

Mid-afternoon _____

Dinner _____

Evening _____

New Foods/Reactions: _____

Stools (amount, number and type): _____

Quick Symptoms Checklist: **Rate Symptoms 0-10**

❑ Headache	❑ Digestive symptoms	Energy level:_____
❑ Joint pain	❑ Abdominal pain	Mood: _____
❑ Muscle pain	❑ Tinnitus	Mental Clarity:_____
❑ Other: _____	❑ Other: _____	Purpose/Hope: _____

My week overall: 0--10

I would describe my week (in one word) as: _____

Because? _____

General progress:

Advanced to a new stage? Y/N   Current stage?_____

New foods tolerated: _____   Foods removed: _____

Animal fats consumed: _____   Avg. daily amount: _____

# of days stock consumed: _____   Avg. daily amount: _____

Probiotics/fermented foods/cultured dairy:

Probiotic supplement: _____Current dose: _____

Die-off symptoms: Y/N   Describe: _____

_____

Beet Kvass _____   Sour Cream _____

Veggie Medley _____   Yogurt _____

Sauerkraut _____   Kefir_____

Detoxing Progress:

# of detox baths: _____ Ingredients: ACV/Epsom/Baking soda

# of days sunbathed: _____ # of minutes per session:_____ minutes

# of days juiced in am: _____ in pm: _____

Ingredients:_____

Overall reactions to detoxing: _____

Symptoms descriptions:

Stools: Daily Y/N   #per day _____   Type(s):_____

Digestion: _____

Mood/energy: _____

Memory/clarity: _____

Sleep/Stress: _____

Typical-for-me symptoms: _____

_____

Date _____

❑ FCLO/HVBO	❑ Probiotic	❑ Detox Bath	❑ AM Juicing	❑ Fat
❑ Omega 3/6	❑ Beet Kvass	❑ Oil Pull	❑ PM Juicing	❑ Stock
❑ Iodine	❑ Milk Kefir	❑ Sunbathing	❑ Movement	❑ Ferments

Take a Moment:

At the end of the day, tell yourself gently: 'I love you, you did the best you could today, and even if you didn't accomplish all you had planned, I love you anyway.' —Anonymous

Tell yourself this tonight. Was it hard?

_____

_____

Today's Focus: _____

Nutritional Intake:

Breakfast _____

Mid-morning_____

Lunch _____

Mid-afternoon _____

Dinner _____

Evening _____

New Foods/Reactions:_____

Stools (amount, number and type): _____

_____

Quick Symptoms Checklist:		**Rate Symptoms 0-10**
❑ Headache	❑ Digestive symptoms	Energy level:_____
❑ Joint pain	❑ Abdominal pain	Mood: _____
❑ Muscle pain	❑ Tinnitus	Mental Clarity: _____
❑ Other: _____	❑ Other: _____	Purpose/Hope: _____

Date _____

❏ FCLO/HVBO	❏ Probiotic	❏ Detox Bath	❏ AM Juicing	❏ Fat
❏ Omega 3/6	❏ Beet Kvass	❏ Oil Pull	❏ PM Juicing	❏ Stock
❏ Iodine	❏ Milk Kefir	❏ Sunbathing	❏ Movement	❏ Ferments

Take a Moment:

And the day came when the risk to remain tight in a bud was more painful than the risk it took to blossom. —Anaïs Nin

Is this today? What risks are you facing?

_____

_____

_____

Today's Focus: _____

Nutritional Intake:

Breakfast _____

Mid-morning_____

Lunch _____

Mid-afternoon _____

Dinner _____

Evening _____

New Foods/Reactions: _____

Stools (amount, number and type): _____

_____

Quick Symptoms Checklist: Rate Symptoms 0-10

❏ Headache	❏ Digestive symptoms	Energy level:_____
❏ Joint pain	❏ Abdominal pain	Mood: _____
❏ Muscle pain	❏ Tinnitus	Mental Clarity: _____
❏ Other: _____	❏ Other: _____	Purpose/Hope: _____

Date _____

❑ FCLO/HVBO	❑ Probiotic	❑ Detox Bath	❑ AM Juicing	❑ Fat
❑ Omega 3/6	❑ Beet Kvass	❑ Oil Pull	❑ PM Juicing	❑ Stock
❑ Iodine	❑ Milk Kefir	❑ Sunbathing	❑ Movement	❑ Ferments

Take a Moment:

I feel the capacity to care is the thing which gives life its deepest significance. —Pablo Casals

What do you care about?

_____

_____

_____

Today's Focus: _____

Nutritional Intake:

Breakfast _____

Mid-morning _____

Lunch _____

Mid-afternoon _____

Dinner _____

Evening _____

New Foods/Reactions: _____

Stools (amount, number and type): _____

_____

Quick Symptoms Checklist:		**Rate Symptoms 0-10**
❑ Headache	❑ Digestive symptoms	Energy level: _____
❑ Joint pain	❑ Abdominal pain	Mood: _____
❑ Muscle pain	❑ Tinnitus	Mental Clarity: _____
❑ Other: _____	❑ Other: _____	Purpose/Hope: _____

Date _____

❏ FCLO/HVBO	❏ Probiotic	❏ Detox Bath	❏ AM Juicing	❏ Fat
❏ Omega 3/6	❏ Beet Kvass	❏ Oil Pull	❏ PM Juicing	❏ Stock
❏ Iodine	❏ Milk Kefir	❏ Sunbathing	❏ Movement	❏ Ferments

Take a Moment:

A good deed is never lost; he who sows courtesy reaps friendship, and he who plants kindness gathers love. —Basil the Great

Where can you plant a kindness today?

_____

_____

Today's Focus: _____

Nutritional Intake:

Breakfast _____

Mid-morning _____

Lunch _____

Mid-afternoon _____

Dinner _____

Evening _____

New Foods/Reactions: _____

Stools (amount, number and type): _____

_____

Quick Symptoms Checklist: Rate Symptoms 0-10

❏ Headache	❏ Digestive symptoms	Energy level: _____
❏ Joint pain	❏ Abdominal pain	Mood: _____
❏ Muscle pain	❏ Tinnitus	Mental Clarity: _____
❏ Other: _____	❏ Other: _____	Purpose/Hope: _____

Date _____

❑ FCLO/HVBO	❑ Probiotic	❑ Detox Bath	❑ AM Juicing	❑ Fat
❑ Omega 3/6	❑ Beet Kvass	❑ Oil Pull	❑ PM Juicing	❑ Stock
❑ Iodine	❑ Milk Kefir	❑ Sunbathing	❑ Movement	❑ Ferments

Take a Moment:

If you are really thankful, what do you do? You share. —W. Clement Stone

What are you thankful for today?

_____

_____

_____

_____

Today's Focus: _____

Nutritional Intake:

Breakfast _____

Mid-morning_____

Lunch _____

Mid-afternoon _____

Dinner _____

Evening _____

New Foods/Reactions:_____

Stools (amount, number and type): _____

Quick Symptoms Checklist: **Rate Symptoms 0-10**

❑ Headache	❑ Digestive symptoms	Energy level:_____
❑ Joint pain	❑ Abdominal pain	Mood: _____
❑ Muscle pain	❑ Tinnitus	Mental Clarity:_____
❑ Other: _____	❑ Other: _____	Purpose/Hope:_____

Date _____

❏ FCLO/HVBO	❏ Probiotic	❏ Detox Bath	❏ AM Juicing	❏ Fat
❏ Omega 3/6	❏ Beet Kvass	❏ Oil Pull	❏ PM Juicing	❏ Stock
❏ Iodine	❏ Milk Kefir	❏ Sunbathing	❏ Movement	❏ Ferments

Take a Moment:

Fear is a reaction, courage is a decision. —Sir Winston Churchill

Is fear your reaction? How can you choose courage today?

_____

_____

_____

_____

Today's Focus: _____

Nutritional Intake:

Breakfast _____

Mid-morning _____

Lunch _____

Mid-afternoon _____

Dinner _____

Evening _____

New Foods/Reactions: _____

Stools (amount, number and type): _____

_____

Quick Symptoms Checklist: Rate Symptoms 0-10

❏ Headache	❏ Digestive symptoms	Energy level:_____
❏ Joint pain	❏ Abdominal pain	Mood: _____
❏ Muscle pain	❏ Tinnitus	Mental Clarity:_____
❏ Other: _____	❏ Other: _____	Purpose/Hope: _____

Date _____

❏ FCLO/HVBO	❏ Probiotic	❏ Detox Bath	❏ AM Juicing	❏ Fat
❏ Omega 3/6	❏ Beet Kvass	❏ Oil Pull	❏ PM Juicing	❏ Stock
❏ Iodine	❏ Milk Kefir	❏ Sunbathing	❏ Movement	❏ Ferments

Take a Moment:

Sharing food with another human being is an intimate act that should not be indulged in lightly. —M.F.K. Fisher

Following GAPS can make it hard to share food with others. Has your heart been able to feel intimate with someone in this way recently?

_____

_____

Today's Focus: _____

Nutritional Intake:

Breakfast _____

Mid-morning_____

Lunch _____

Mid-afternoon _____

Dinner _____

Evening _____

New Foods/Reactions: _____

Stools (amount, number and type): _____

Quick Symptoms Checklist: **Rate Symptoms 0-10**

❏ Headache	❏ Digestive symptoms	Energy level:_____
❏ Joint pain	❏ Abdominal pain	Mood: _____
❏ Muscle pain	❏ Tinnitus	Mental Clarity: _____
❏ Other: _____	❏ Other: _____	Purpose/Hope: _____

My week overall: 0--10

I would describe my week (in one word) as: _____

Because? _____

General progress:

Advanced to a new stage? Y/N   Current stage?_____

New foods tolerated: _____   Foods removed: _____

Animal fats consumed: _____   Avg. daily amount: _____

# of days stock consumed: _____   Avg. daily amount: _____

Probiotics/fermented foods/cultured dairy:

Probiotic supplement: _____Current dose: _____

Die-off symptoms: Y/N   Describe: _____

_____

Beet Kvass _____   Sour Cream _____

Veggie Medley_____   Yogurt _____

Sauerkraut_____   Kefir_____

Detoxing Progress:

# of detox baths: _____ Ingredients: ACV/Epsom/Baking soda

# of days sunbathed: _____ # of minutes per session:_____ minutes

# of days juiced in am: _____in pm: _____

Ingredients:_____

Overall reactions to detoxing: _____

Symptoms descriptions:

Stools: Daily Y/N   #per day _____   Type(s):_____

Digestion: _____

Mood/energy: _____

Memory/clarity: _____

Sleep/Stress: _____

Typical-for-me symptoms: _____

_____

Date _____

❏ FCLO/HVBO	❏ Probiotic	❏ Detox Bath	❏ AM Juicing	❏ Fat
❏ Omega 3/6	❏ Beet Kvass	❏ Oil Pull	❏ PM Juicing	❏ Stock
❏ Iodine	❏ Milk Kefir	❏ Sunbathing	❏ Movement	❏ Ferments

Take a Moment:

Hardships often prepare ordinary people for an extrodinary destiny.
—C.S. Lewis

What do you think your hardships may be preparing you for?

_____

_____

_____

Today's Focus: _____

Nutritional Intake:

Breakfast _____

Mid-morning _____

Lunch _____

Mid-afternoon _____

Dinner _____

Evening _____

New Foods/Reactions: _____

Stools (amount, number and type): _____

Quick Symptoms Checklist: **Rate Symptoms 0-10**

❏ Headache	❏ Digestive symptoms	Energy level:_____
❏ Joint pain	❏ Abdominal pain	Mood: _____
❏ Muscle pain	❏ Tinnitus	Mental Clarity: _____
❏ Other: _____	❏ Other: _____	Purpose/Hope: _____

Date _____

- ❏ FCLO/HVBO
- ❏ Omega 3/6
- ❏ Iodine
- ❏ Probiotic
- ❏ Beet Kvass
- ❏ Milk Kefir
- ❏ Detox Bath
- ❏ Oil Pull
- ❏ Sunbathing
- ❏ AM Juicing
- ❏ PM Juicing
- ❏ Movement
- ❏ Fat
- ❏ Stock
- ❏ Ferments

Take a Moment:

Just like there's always time for pain, there's always time for healing.
—Jennifer Brown

Are you impatient for healing to happen?

_____

_____

_____

Today's Focus: _____

Nutritional Intake:

Breakfast _____

Mid-morning_____

Lunch _____

Mid-afternoon _____

Dinner _____

Evening _____

New Foods/Reactions: _____

Stools (amount, number and type): _____

_____

Quick Symptoms Checklist: Rate Symptoms 0-10

❏ Headache	❏ Digestive symptoms	Energy level:_____
❏ Joint pain	❏ Abdominal pain	Mood: _____
❏ Muscle pain	❏ Tinnitus	Mental Clarity: _____
❏ Other: _____	❏ Other: _____	Purpose/Hope: _____

Date _____

❏ FCLO/HVBO	❏ Probiotic	❏ Detox Bath	❏ AM Juicing	❏ Fat
❏ Omega 3/6	❏ Beet Kvass	❏ Oil Pull	❏ PM Juicing	❏ Stock
❏ Iodine	❏ Milk Kefir	❏ Sunbathing	❏ Movement	❏ Ferments

Take a Moment:

The sun shall always rise upon a new day and there shall always be a rose garden within me. Yes, there is a part of me that is broken, but my broken soil gives way to my wild roses. —C. JoyBell C.

What beautiful roses do you see in you today?

_____

_____

_____

Today's Focus: _____

Nutritional Intake:

Breakfast _____

Mid-morning _____

Lunch _____

Mid-afternoon _____

Dinner _____

Evening _____

New Foods/Reactions: _____

Stools (amount, number and type): _____

Quick Symptoms Checklist: **Rate Symptoms 0-10**

❏ Headache	❏ Digestive symptoms	Energy level:_____
❏ Joint pain	❏ Abdominal pain	Mood: _____
❏ Muscle pain	❏ Tinnitus	Mental Clarity:_____
❏ Other: _____	❏ Other: _____	Purpose/Hope: _____

Date _____

Take a Moment:

Boredom is the feeling that everything is a waste of time; serenity, that nothing is. —Thomas Szaza

Are you feeling bored? How can you switch your thinking?

_____

_____

_____

Today's Focus: _____

Nutritional Intake:

Breakfast _____

Mid-morning_____

Lunch _____

Mid-afternoon _____

Dinner _____

Evening _____

New Foods/Reactions: _____

Stools (amount, number and type): _____

Quick Symptoms Checklist: Rate Symptoms 0-10

❏ Headache	❏ Digestive symptoms	Energy level:_____
❏ Joint pain	❏ Abdominal pain	Mood: _____
❏ Muscle pain	❏ Tinnitus	Mental Clarity: _____
❏ Other: _____	❏ Other: _____	Purpose/Hope: _____

Date _____

❏ FCLO/HVBO	❏ Probiotic	❏ Detox Bath	❏ AM Juicing	❏ Fat
❏ Omega 3/6	❏ Beet Kvass	❏ Oil Pull	❏ PM Juicing	❏ Stock
❏ Iodine	❏ Milk Kefir	❏ Sunbathing	❏ Movement	❏ Ferments

Take a Moment:

It's harder to heal than it is to kill. —Tamora Pierce

Do you feel like you would rather give up than keep healing?

_____

_____

_____

_____

Today's Focus: _____

Nutritional Intake:

Breakfast _____

Mid-morning_____

Lunch _____

Mid-afternoon _____

Dinner _____

Evening _____

New Foods/Reactions: _____

Stools (amount, number and type): _____

Quick Symptoms Checklist: Rate Symptoms 0-10

❏ Headache	❏ Digestive symptoms	Energy level:_____
❏ Joint pain	❏ Abdominal pain	Mood: _____
❏ Muscle pain	❏ Tinnitus	Mental Clarity: _____
❏ Other: _____	❏ Other: _____	Purpose/Hope: _____

Date _____

❑ FCLO/HVBO	❑ Probiotic	❑ Detox Bath	❑ AM Juicing	❑ Fat
❑ Omega 3/6	❑ Beet Kvass	❑ Oil Pull	❑ PM Juicing	❑ Stock
❑ Iodine	❑ Milk Kefir	❑ Sunbathing	❑ Movement	❑ Ferments

Take a Moment:

The crisis of today is the joke of tomorrow. —H.G.Wells

Write about a past crisis that you laugh about now.

_____

_____

_____

_____

Today's Focus: _____

Nutritional Intake:

Breakfast _____

Mid-morning _____

Lunch _____

Mid-afternoon _____

Dinner _____

Evening _____

New Foods/Reactions: _____

Stools (amount, number and type): _____

_____

Quick Symptoms Checklist: Rate Symptoms 0-10

❑ Headache	❑ Digestive symptoms	Energy level:_____
❑ Joint pain	❑ Abdominal pain	Mood: _____
❑ Muscle pain	❑ Tinnitus	Mental Clarity:_____
❑ Other: _____	❑ Other: _____	Purpose/Hope: _____

Date _____

❏ FCLO/HVBO	❏ Probiotic	❏ Detox Bath	❏ AM Juicing	❏ Fat
❏ Omega 3/6	❏ Beet Kvass	❏ Oil Pull	❏ PM Juicing	❏ Stock
❏ Iodine	❏ Milk Kefir	❏ Sunbathing	❏ Movement	❏ Ferments

Take a Moment:

The best remedy for those who are afraid, lonely, or unhappy is to go outside, somewhere where they can be quiet, alone with the heavens, nature, and God. Because only then does one feel that all is as it should be and that God wishes to see people happy, amidst the simple beauty of nature. —Anne Frank

Make a plan to get alone in nature, soon!

_____

_____

Today's Focus: _____

Nutritional Intake:

Breakfast _____

Mid-morning_____

Lunch _____

Mid-afternoon _____

Dinner _____

Evening _____

New Foods/Reactions:_____

Stools (amount, number and type): _____

_____

Quick Symptoms Checklist: Rate Symptoms 0-10

❏ Headache	❏ Digestive symptoms	Energy level:_____
❏ Joint pain	❏ Abdominal pain	Mood: _____
❏ Muscle pain	❏ Tinnitus	Mental Clarity: _____
❏ Other: _____	❏ Other: _____	Purpose/Hope: _____

My week overall: 0--10

I would describe my week (in one word) as: _____

Because? _____

General progress:

Advanced to a new stage? Y/N   Current stage?_____

New foods tolerated: _____   Foods removed: _____

Animal fats consumed:_____   Avg. daily amount: _____

# of days stock consumed: _____   Avg. daily amount: _____

Probiotics/fermented foods/cultured dairy:

Probiotic supplement: _____Current dose: _____

Die-off symptoms: Y/N   Describe: _____

_____

Beet Kvass_____   Sour Cream_____

Veggie Medley_____   Yogurt _____

Sauerkraut_____   Kefir_____

Detoxing Progress:

# of detox baths: _____ Ingredients: ACV/Epsom/Baking soda

# of days sunbathed: _____ # of minutes per session:_____ minutes

# of days juiced in am: _____in pm: _____

Ingredients:_____

Overall reactions to detoxing: _____

Symptoms descriptions:

Stools: Daily Y/N   #per day _____   Type(s):_____

Digestion: _____

Mood/energy: _____

Memory/clarity: _____

Sleep/Stress: _____

Typical-for-me symptoms: _____

_____

Date _____

❑ FCLO/HVBO	❑ Probiotic	❑ Detox Bath	❑ AM Juicing	❑ Fat
❑ Omega 3/6	❑ Beet Kvass	❑ Oil Pull	❑ PM Juicing	❑ Stock
❑ Iodine	❑ Milk Kefir	❑ Sunbathing	❑ Movement	❑ Ferments

Take a Moment:

Do not let making a living prevent you from making a life.
—John R. Wooden

Slow down and live today.

_____

_____

_____

Today's Focus: _____

Nutritional Intake:

Breakfast _____

Mid-morning_____

Lunch _____

Mid-afternoon _____

Dinner _____

Evening _____

New Foods/Reactions: _____

Stools (amount, number and type): _____

_____

Quick Symptoms Checklist: **Rate Symptoms 0-10**

❑ Headache	❑ Digestive symptoms	Energy level:_____
❑ Joint pain	❑ Abdominal pain	Mood: _____
❑ Muscle pain	❑ Tinnitus	Mental Clarity: _____
❑ Other: _____	❑ Other: _____	Purpose/Hope: _____

Date _____

❑ FCLO/HVBO	❑ Probiotic	❑ Detox Bath	❑ AM Juicing	❑ Fat
❑ Omega 3/6	❑ Beet Kvass	❑ Oil Pull	❑ PM Juicing	❑ Stock
❑ Iodine	❑ Milk Kefir	❑ Sunbathing	❑ Movement	❑ Ferments

Take a Moment:

How we spend our days is, of course, how we spend our lives.
—Annie Dillard

Each day is a new chance to spend our life differently. Write down one way you want to spend today.

_____

_____

_____

Today's Focus: _____

Nutritional Intake:

Breakfast _____

Mid-morning _____

Lunch _____

Mid-afternoon _____

Dinner _____

Evening _____

New Foods/Reactions: _____

Stools (amount, number and type): _____

_____

Quick Symptoms Checklist: **Rate Symptoms 0-10**

❑ Headache	❑ Digestive symptoms	Energy level:_____
❑ Joint pain	❑ Abdominal pain	Mood: _____
❑ Muscle pain	❑ Tinnitus	Mental Clarity: _____
❑ Other: _____	❑ Other: _____	Purpose/Hope: _____

Date _____

❑ FCLO/HVBO	❑ Probiotic	❑ Detox Bath	❑ AM Juicing	❑ Fat
❑ Omega 3/6	❑ Beet Kvass	❑ Oil Pull	❑ PM Juicing	❑ Stock
❑ Iodine	❑ Milk Kefir	❑ Sunbathing	❑ Movement	❑ Ferments

Take a Moment:

Listening, not imitation, may be the sincerest form of flattery.
—Dr. Joyce Brothers

Have you been blessed by someone doing something for you? Who could you listen to today?

_____

_____

_____

Today's Focus: _____

Nutritional Intake:

Breakfast _____

Mid-morning_____

Lunch _____

Mid-afternoon _____

Dinner _____

Evening _____

New Foods/Reactions: _____

Stools (amount, number and type): _____

Quick Symptoms Checklist: **Rate Symptoms 0-10**

Quick Symptoms Checklist		Rate Symptoms 0-10
❑ Headache	❑ Digestive symptoms	Energy level:_____
❑ Joint pain	❑ Abdominal pain	Mood: _____
❑ Muscle pain	❑ Tinnitus	Mental Clarity: _____
❑ Other: _____	❑ Other: _____	Purpose/Hope: _____

Date _____

❏ FCLO/HVBO	❏ Probiotic	❏ Detox Bath	❏ AM Juicing	❏ Fat
❏ Omega 3/6	❏ Beet Kvass	❏ Oil Pull	❏ PM Juicing	❏ Stock
❏ Iodine	❏ Milk Kefir	❏ Sunbathing	❏ Movement	❏ Ferments

Take a Moment:

Patience is the companion of wisdom. —St. Augustine

How do you think you will need to practice patience today?

_____

_____

_____

_____

Today's Focus: _____

Nutritional Intake:

Breakfast _____

Mid-morning_____

Lunch _____

Mid-afternoon _____

Dinner _____

Evening _____

New Foods/Reactions: _____

Stools (amount, number and type): _____

_____

Quick Symptoms Checklist: **Rate Symptoms 0-10**

❏ Headache	❏ Digestive symptoms	Energy level:_____
❏ Joint pain	❏ Abdominal pain	Mood: _____
❏ Muscle pain	❏ Tinnitus	Mental Clarity: _____
❏ Other: _____	❏ Other: _____	Purpose/Hope: _____

Date _____

❏ FCLO/HVBO	❏ Probiotic	❏ Detox Bath	❏ AM Juicing	❏ Fat
❏ Omega 3/6	❏ Beet Kvass	❏ Oil Pull	❏ PM Juicing	❏ Stock
❏ Iodine	❏ Milk Kefir	❏ Sunbathing	❏ Movement	❏ Ferments

Take a Moment:

It is terrible to destroy a person's picture of himself in the interests of truth or some other abstraction. —Doris Lessing

It's natural to want people to think like us. But which is more important, the person, or the thought?

_____

_____

_____

Today's Focus: _____

Nutritional Intake:

Breakfast _____

Mid-morning_____

Lunch _____

Mid-afternoon _____

Dinner _____

Evening _____

New Foods/Reactions:_____

Stools (amount, number and type): _____

Quick Symptoms Checklist: **Rate Symptoms 0-10**

❏ Headache	❏ Digestive symptoms	Energy level:_____
❏ Joint pain	❏ Abdominal pain	Mood: _____
❏ Muscle pain	❏ Tinnitus	Mental Clarity: _____
❏ Other: _____	❏ Other: _____	Purpose/Hope: _____

Date _____

❏ FCLO/HVBO	❏ Probiotic	❏ Detox Bath	❏ AM Juicing	❏ Fat
❏ Omega 3/6	❏ Beet Kvass	❏ Oil Pull	❏ PM Juicing	❏ Stock
❏ Iodine	❏ Milk Kefir	❏ Sunbathing	❏ Movement	❏ Ferments

Take a Moment:

Tact is the knack of making a point without making an enemy.
—Sir Isaac Newton

Health is a volitile topic. When talking to others, how do you use tact?

_____

_____

_____

Today's Focus: _____

Nutritional Intake:

Breakfast _____

Mid-morning_____

Lunch _____

Mid-afternoon _____

Dinner _____

Evening _____

New Foods/Reactions: _____

Stools (amount, number and type): _____

_____

Quick Symptoms Checklist: **Rate Symptoms 0-10**

❏ Headache	❏ Digestive symptoms	Energy level:_____
❏ Joint pain	❏ Abdominal pain	Mood: _____
❏ Muscle pain	❏ Tinnitus	Mental Clarity: _____
❏ Other: _____	❏ Other: _____	Purpose/Hope: _____

Date _____

❏ FCLO/HVBO	❏ Probiotic	❏ Detox Bath	❏ AM Juicing	❏ Fat
❏ Omega 3/6	❏ Beet Kvass	❏ Oil Pull	❏ PM Juicing	❏ Stock
❏ Iodine	❏ Milk Kefir	❏ Sunbathing	❏ Movement	❏ Ferments

Take a Moment:

I am not this hair, I am not this skin, I am the soul that lives within.
—Rumi

When we focus on health, this can get lost. Focus on your soul today.

_____

_____

_____

Today's Focus: _____

Nutritional Intake:

Breakfast _____

Mid-morning _____

Lunch _____

Mid-afternoon _____

Dinner _____

Evening _____

New Foods/Reactions: _____

Stools (amount, number and type): _____

Quick Symptoms Checklist: **Rate Symptoms 0-10**

❏ Headache	❏ Digestive symptoms	Energy level:_____
❏ Joint pain	❏ Abdominal pain	Mood: _____
❏ Muscle pain	❏ Tinnitus	Mental Clarity: _____
❏ Other: _____	❏ Other: _____	Purpose/Hope: _____

My week overall: 0--10

I would describe my week (in one word) as: _____

Because? _____

General progress:

Advanced to a new stage? Y/N   Current stage?_____

New foods tolerated: _____   Foods removed: _____

Animal fats consumed: _____   Avg. daily amount: _____

# of days stock consumed: _____   Avg. daily amount: _____

Probiotics/fermented foods/cultured dairy:

Probiotic supplement: _____Current dose: _____

Die-off symptoms: Y/N   Describe: _____

_____

Beet Kvass _____   Sour Cream _____

Veggie Medley_____   Yogurt _____

Sauerkraut_____   Kefir_____

Detoxing Progress:

# of detox baths: _____ Ingredients: ACV/Epsom/Baking soda

# of days sunbathed: _____ # of minutes per session:_____ minutes

# of days juiced in am: _____in pm: _____

Ingredients:_____

Overall reactions to detoxing: _____

Symptoms descriptions:

Stools: Daily Y/N   #per day _____   Type(s):_____

Digestion: _____

Mood/energy: _____

Memory/clarity: _____

Sleep/Stress: _____

Typical-for-me symptoms: _____

_____

Date _____

❏ FCLO/HVBO	❏ Probiotic	❏ Detox Bath	❏ AM Juicing	❏ Fat
❏ Omega 3/6	❏ Beet Kvass	❏ Oil Pull	❏ PM Juicing	❏ Stock
❏ Iodine	❏ Milk Kefir	❏ Sunbathing	❏ Movement	❏ Ferments

Take a Moment:

First, keep the peace within yourself, then you can also bring peace to others. —Thomas A Kempis

Plan a time to focus on being calm and peaceful today.

_____

_____

_____

Today's Focus: _____

Nutritional Intake:

Breakfast _____

Mid-morning _____

Lunch _____

Mid-afternoon _____

Dinner _____

Evening _____

New Foods/Reactions: _____

Stools (amount, number and type): _____

_____

Quick Symptoms Checklist: Rate Symptoms 0-10

❏ Headache	❏ Digestive symptoms	Energy level:_____
❏ Joint pain	❏ Abdominal pain	Mood: _____
❏ Muscle pain	❏ Tinnitus	Mental Clarity: _____
❏ Other: _____	❏ Other: _____	Purpose/Hope: _____

Date _____

❑ FCLO/HVBO	❑ Probiotic	❑ Detox Bath	❑ AM Juicing	❑ Fat
❑ Omega 3/6	❑ Beet Kvass	❑ Oil Pull	❑ PM Juicing	❑ Stock
❑ Iodine	❑ Milk Kefir	❑ Sunbathing	❑ Movement	❑ Ferments

Take a Moment:

Character consists of what you do on the third and fourth tries.
—James Michener

Do you feel like you have to keep trying?
What will you do with this try?

_____

_____

_____

Today's Focus: _____

Nutritional Intake:

Breakfast _____

Mid-morning _____

Lunch _____

Mid-afternoon _____

Dinner _____

Evening _____

New Foods/Reactions: _____

Stools (amount, number and type): _____

_____

Quick Symptoms Checklist: Rate Symptoms 0-10

❑ Headache	❑ Digestive symptoms	Energy level:_____
❑ Joint pain	❑ Abdominal pain	Mood: _____
❑ Muscle pain	❑ Tinnitus	Mental Clarity:_____
❑ Other: _____	❑ Other: _____	Purpose/Hope: _____

Date _____

❑ FCLO/HVBO	❑ Probiotic	❑ Detox Bath	❑ AM Juicing	❑ Fat
❑ Omega 3/6	❑ Beet Kvass	❑ Oil Pull	❑ PM Juicing	❑ Stock
❑ Iodine	❑ Milk Kefir	❑ Sunbathing	❑ Movement	❑ Ferments

Take a Moment:

Joy is a net of love in which you can catch souls. —Mother Teresa

Can you have joy today?

_____

_____

_____

_____

Today's Focus: _____

Nutritional Intake:

Breakfast _____

Mid-morning _____

Lunch _____

Mid-afternoon _____

Dinner _____

Evening _____

New Foods/Reactions: _____

Stools (amount, number and type): _____

Quick Symptoms Checklist: **Rate Symptoms 0-10**

❑ Headache	❑ Digestive symptoms	Energy level: _____
❑ Joint pain	❑ Abdominal pain	Mood: _____
❑ Muscle pain	❑ Tinnitus	Mental Clarity: _____
❑ Other: _____	❑ Other: _____	Purpose/Hope: _____

Date _____

❑ FCLO/HVBO	❑ Probiotic	❑ Detox Bath	❑ AM Juicing	❑ Fat
❑ Omega 3/6	❑ Beet Kvass	❑ Oil Pull	❑ PM Juicing	❑ Stock
❑ Iodine	❑ Milk Kefir	❑ Sunbathing	❑ Movement	❑ Ferments

Take a Moment:

If you do not tell the truth about yourself,
you cannot tell it about other people. —Virginia Woolf

Are you truthful with yourself?

_____

_____

_____

Today's Focus: _____

Nutritional Intake:

Breakfast _____

Mid-morning _____

Lunch _____

Mid-afternoon _____

Dinner _____

Evening _____

New Foods/Reactions: _____

Stools (amount, number and type): _____

_____

Quick Symptoms Checklist: **Rate Symptoms 0-10**

❑ Headache	❑ Digestive symptoms	Energy level:_____
❑ Joint pain	❑ Abdominal pain	Mood: _____
❑ Muscle pain	❑ Tinnitus	Mental Clarity: _____
❑ Other: _____	❑ Other: _____	Purpose/Hope: _____

Date _____

❏ FCLO/HVBO	❏ Probiotic	❏ Detox Bath	❏ AM Juicing	❏ Fat
❏ Omega 3/6	❏ Beet Kvass	❏ Oil Pull	❏ PM Juicing	❏ Stock
❏ Iodine	❏ Milk Kefir	❏ Sunbathing	❏ Movement	❏ Ferments

Take a Moment:

If a fellow isn't thankful for what he's got, he isn't likely to be thankful for what he's going to get. —Frank A. Clark

How can you choose to be a little more thankful today?

_____

_____

_____

Today's Focus: _____

Nutritional Intake:

Breakfast _____

Mid-morning_____

Lunch _____

Mid-afternoon _____

Dinner _____

Evening _____

New Foods/Reactions: _____

Stools (amount, number and type): _____

_____

Quick Symptoms Checklist: Rate Symptoms 0-10

❏ Headache	❏ Digestive symptoms	Energy level:_____
❏ Joint pain	❏ Abdominal pain	Mood: _____
❏ Muscle pain	❏ Tinnitus	Mental Clarity: _____
❏ Other: _____	❏ Other: _____	Purpose/Hope: _____

Date _____

❏ FCLO/HVBO	❏ Probiotic	❏ Detox Bath	❏ AM Juicing	❏ Fat
❏ Omega 3/6	❏ Beet Kvass	❏ Oil Pull	❏ PM Juicing	❏ Stock
❏ Iodine	❏ Milk Kefir	❏ Sunbathing	❏ Movement	❏ Ferments

Take a Moment:

Never tell people how to do things. Tell them what to do and they will surprise you with their ingenuity. —General George S Patton

What is something you figured out how to do well? If you would like, share it!

_____

_____

_____

Today's Focus: _____

Nutritional Intake:

Breakfast _____

Mid-morning _____

Lunch _____

Mid-afternoon _____

Dinner _____

Evening _____

New Foods/Reactions: _____

Stools (amount, number and type): _____

Quick Symptoms Checklist: **Rate Symptoms 0-10**

❏ Headache	❏ Digestive symptoms	Energy level:_____
❏ Joint pain	❏ Abdominal pain	Mood: _____
❏ Muscle pain	❏ Tinnitus	Mental Clarity: _____
❏ Other: _____	❏ Other: _____	Purpose/Hope: _____

Date _____

❏ FCLO/HVBO	❏ Probiotic	❏ Detox Bath	❏ AM Juicing	❏ Fat
❏ Omega 3/6	❏ Beet Kvass	❏ Oil Pull	❏ PM Juicing	❏ Stock
❏ Iodine	❏ Milk Kefir	❏ Sunbathing	❏ Movement	❏ Ferments

Take a Moment:

In summer, the song sings itself. —William Carlos Williams

Make a plan to be outside, enjoying the summer!

_____

_____

_____

_____

Today's Focus: _____

Nutritional Intake:

Breakfast _____

Mid-morning_____

Lunch _____

Mid-afternoon _____

Dinner _____

Evening _____

New Foods/Reactions:_____

Stools (amount, number and type): _____

Quick Symptoms Checklist: **Rate Symptoms 0-10**

❏ Headache	❏ Digestive symptoms	Energy level:_____
❏ Joint pain	❏ Abdominal pain	Mood: _____
❏ Muscle pain	❏ Tinnitus	Mental Clarity: _____
❏ Other: _____	❏ Other: _____	Purpose/Hope: _____

My week overall: 0--10

I would describe my week (in one word) as: _____

Because? _____

General progress:

Advanced to a new stage? Y/N   Current stage?_____

New foods tolerated: _____   Foods removed: _____

Animal fats consumed: _____   Avg. daily amount: _____

# of days stock consumed: _____   Avg. daily amount: _____

Probiotics/fermented foods/cultured dairy:

Probiotic supplement: _____Current dose: _____

Die-off symptoms: Y/N   Describe: _____

_____

Beet Kvass _____   Sour Cream _____

Veggie Medley_____   Yogurt _____

Sauerkraut_____   Kefir_____

Detoxing Progress:

# of detox baths: _____ Ingredients: ACV/Epsom/Baking soda

# of days sunbathed: _____ # of minutes per session:_____ minutes

# of days juiced in am: _____in pm: _____

Ingredients:_____

Overall reactions to detoxing: _____

Symptoms descriptions:

Stools: Daily Y/N   #per day _____   Type(s):_____

Digestion: _____

Mood/energy: _____

Memory/clarity: _____

Sleep/Stress: _____

Typical-for-me symptoms: _____

_____

Date _____

❑ FCLO/HVBO	❑ Probiotic	❑ Detox Bath	❑ AM Juicing	❑ Fat
❑ Omega 3/6	❑ Beet Kvass	❑ Oil Pull	❑ PM Juicing	❑ Stock
❑ Iodine	❑ Milk Kefir	❑ Sunbathing	❑ Movement	❑ Ferments

Take a Moment:

Study the past, if you would divine the future. —Confucius

Look back. What can you learn from the past?

_____

_____

_____

_____

Today's Focus: _____

Nutritional Intake:

Breakfast _____

Mid-morning_____

Lunch _____

Mid-afternoon _____

Dinner _____

Evening _____

New Foods/Reactions: _____

Stools (amount, number and type): _____

Quick Symptoms Checklist: Rate Symptoms 0-10

❑ Headache	❑ Digestive symptoms	Energy level:_____
❑ Joint pain	❑ Abdominal pain	Mood: _____
❑ Muscle pain	❑ Tinnitus	Mental Clarity: _____
❑ Other: _____	❑ Other: _____	Purpose/Hope: _____

Date _____

❑ FCLO/HVBO	❑ Probiotic	❑ Detox Bath	❑ AM Juicing	❑ Fat
❑ Omega 3/6	❑ Beet Kvass	❑ Oil Pull	❑ PM Juicing	❑ Stock
❑ Iodine	❑ Milk Kefir	❑ Sunbathing	❑ Movement	❑ Ferments

Take a Moment:

You've been criticising yourself for years and it hasn't worked. Try approving of yourself and see what happens. —Louise L. Hay

Write down 5 things that you like about yourself.

_____

_____

_____

Today's Focus: _____

Nutritional Intake:

Breakfast _____

Mid-morning_____

Lunch _____

Mid-afternoon _____

Dinner _____

Evening _____

New Foods/Reactions:_____

Stools (amount, number and type): _____

_____

Quick Symptoms Checklist: Rate Symptoms 0-10

❑ Headache	❑ Digestive symptoms	Energy level:_____
❑ Joint pain	❑ Abdominal pain	Mood: _____
❑ Muscle pain	❑ Tinnitus	Mental Clarity:_____
❑ Other: _____	❑ Other: _____	Purpose/Hope: _____

Date _____

❏ FCLO/HVBO	❏ Probiotic	❏ Detox Bath	❏ AM Juicing	❏ Fat
❏ Omega 3/6	❏ Beet Kvass	❏ Oil Pull	❏ PM Juicing	❏ Stock
❏ Iodine	❏ Milk Kefir	❏ Sunbathing	❏ Movement	❏ Ferments

Take a Moment:

It's true that laughter really is cheap medicine. It's a prescription anyone can afford. And best of all, you can fill it right now.
—Steve Goodier

How can you fill your "prescription" today?

_____

_____

_____

Today's Focus: _____

Nutritional Intake:

Breakfast _____

Mid-morning _____

Lunch _____

Mid-afternoon _____

Dinner _____

Evening _____

New Foods/Reactions: _____

Stools (amount, number and type): _____

_____

Quick Symptoms Checklist:　　　　　**Rate Symptoms 0-10**

❏ Headache	❏ Digestive symptoms	Energy level: _____
❏ Joint pain	❏ Abdominal pain	Mood: _____
❏ Muscle pain	❏ Tinnitus	Mental Clarity: _____
❏ Other: _____	❏ Other: _____	Purpose/Hope: _____

Date _____

❑ FCLO/HVBO	❑ Probiotic	❑ Detox Bath	❑ AM Juicing	❑ Fat
❑ Omega 3/6	❑ Beet Kvass	❑ Oil Pull	❑ PM Juicing	❑ Stock
❑ Iodine	❑ Milk Kefir	❑ Sunbathing	❑ Movement	❑ Ferments

Take a Moment:

When we cannot get what we love, we must love what is within our reach. —French Proverb

What is within your reach? Write about what you love about it.

_____

_____

_____

Today's Focus: _____

Nutritional Intake:

Breakfast _____

Mid-morning_____

Lunch _____

Mid-afternoon _____

Dinner _____

Evening _____

New Foods/Reactions:_____

Stools (amount, number and type): _____

_____

Quick Symptoms Checklist: **Rate Symptoms 0-10**

❑ Headache	❑ Digestive symptoms	Energy level:_____
❑ Joint pain	❑ Abdominal pain	Mood: _____
❑ Muscle pain	❑ Tinnitus	Mental Clarity: _____
❑ Other: _____	❑ Other: _____	Purpose/Hope: _____

Date _____

❑ FCLO/HVBO	❑ Probiotic	❑ Detox Bath	❑ AM Juicing	❑ Fat
❑ Omega 3/6	❑ Beet Kvass	❑ Oil Pull	❑ PM Juicing	❑ Stock
❑ Iodine	❑ Milk Kefir	❑ Sunbathing	❑ Movement	❑ Ferments

Take a Moment:

You just can't beat the person who never gives up. —Babe Ruth

Do you feel like you can keep going again today?

_____

_____

_____

_____

Today's Focus: _____

Nutritional Intake:

Breakfast _____

Mid-morning_____

Lunch _____

Mid-afternoon _____

Dinner _____

Evening _____

New Foods/Reactions: _____

Stools (amount, number and type): _____

Quick Symptoms Checklist: **Rate Symptoms 0-10**

❑ Headache	❑ Digestive symptoms	Energy level:_____
❑ Joint pain	❑ Abdominal pain	Mood: _____
❑ Muscle pain	❑ Tinnitus	Mental Clarity: _____
❑ Other: _____	❑ Other: _____	Purpose/Hope: _____

Date _____

❏ FCLO/HVBO	❏ Probiotic	❏ Detox Bath	❏ AM Juicing	❏ Fat
❏ Omega 3/6	❏ Beet Kvass	❏ Oil Pull	❏ PM Juicing	❏ Stock
❏ Iodine	❏ Milk Kefir	❏ Sunbathing	❏ Movement	❏ Ferments

Take a Moment:

The two enemies of human happiness are pain and boredom.
—Arthur Schopenhauer

Are you fighting with one of these enemies today?

_____

_____

_____

Today's Focus: _____

Nutritional Intake:

Breakfast _____

Mid-morning _____

Lunch _____

Mid-afternoon _____

Dinner _____

Evening _____

New Foods/Reactions: _____

Stools (amount, number and type): _____

_____

Quick Symptoms Checklist: **Rate Symptoms 0-10**

❏ Headache	❏ Digestive symptoms	Energy level: _____
❏ Joint pain	❏ Abdominal pain	Mood: _____
❏ Muscle pain	❏ Tinnitus	Mental Clarity: _____
❏ Other: _____	❏ Other: _____	Purpose/Hope: _____

Date _____

❏ FCLO/HVBO	❏ Probiotic	❏ Detox Bath	❏ AM Juicing	❏ Fat
❏ Omega 3/6	❏ Beet Kvass	❏ Oil Pull	❏ PM Juicing	❏ Stock
❏ Iodine	❏ Milk Kefir	❏ Sunbathing	❏ Movement	❏ Ferments

Take a Moment:

> *In the days that follow, I discover that anger is easier to handle than grief.* —Emily Giffin

Do you find yourself getting angry often?
Do you think you are ignoring some grief?

_____

_____

_____

Today's Focus: _____

Nutritional Intake:

Breakfast _____

Mid-morning _____

Lunch _____

Mid-afternoon _____

Dinner _____

Evening _____

New Foods/Reactions: _____

Stools (amount, number and type): _____

Quick Symptoms Checklist: **Rate Symptoms 0-10**

Quick Symptoms Checklist		Rate Symptoms 0-10
❏ Headache	❏ Digestive symptoms	Energy level:_____
❏ Joint pain	❏ Abdominal pain	Mood: _____
❏ Muscle pain	❏ Tinnitus	Mental Clarity: _____
❏ Other: _____	❏ Other: _____	Purpose/Hope: _____

My week overall: 0---10

I would describe my week (in one word) as: _____

Because? _____

General progress:

Advanced to a new stage? Y/N   Current stage?_____

New foods tolerated: _____   Foods removed: _____

Animal fats consumed: _____   Avg. daily amount: _____

# of days stock consumed: _____   Avg. daily amount: _____

Probiotics/fermented foods/cultured dairy:

Probiotic supplement: _____ Current dose: _____

Die-off symptoms: Y/N   Describe: _____

_____

Beet Kvass _____   Sour Cream _____

Veggie Medley _____   Yogurt _____

Sauerkraut _____   Kefir _____

Detoxing Progress:

# of detox baths: _____ Ingredients: ACV/Epsom/Baking soda

# of days sunbathed: _____ # of minutes per session:_____ minutes

# of days juiced in am: _____ in pm: _____

Ingredients:_____

Overall reactions to detoxing: _____

Symptoms descriptions:

Stools: Daily Y/N   #per day _____   Type(s):_____

Digestion: _____

Mood/energy: _____

Memory/clarity: _____

Sleep/Stress: _____

Typical-for-me symptoms: _____

_____

Date _____

❏ FCLO/HVBO	❏ Probiotic	❏ Detox Bath	❏ AM Juicing	❏ Fat
❏ Omega 3/6	❏ Beet Kvass	❏ Oil Pull	❏ PM Juicing	❏ Stock
❏ Iodine	❏ Milk Kefir	❏ Sunbathing	❏ Movement	❏ Ferments

Take a Moment:

Man, when he does not grieve, hardly exists. —Antonio Porchia

Take time to grieve about what you wrote down yesterday.

_____

_____

_____

Today's Focus: _____

Nutritional Intake:

Breakfast _____

Mid-morning_____

Lunch _____

Mid-afternoon _____

Dinner _____

Evening _____

New Foods/Reactions: _____

Stools (amount, number and type): _____

_____

Quick Symptoms Checklist: **Rate Symptoms 0-10**

❏ Headache	❏ Digestive symptoms	Energy level:_____
❏ Joint pain	❏ Abdominal pain	Mood: _____
❏ Muscle pain	❏ Tinnitus	Mental Clarity: _____
❏ Other: _____	❏ Other: _____	Purpose/Hope: _____

Date _____

❑ FCLO/HVBO	❑ Probiotic	❑ Detox Bath	❑ AM Juicing	❑ Fat
❑ Omega 3/6	❑ Beet Kvass	❑ Oil Pull	❑ PM Juicing	❑ Stock
❑ Iodine	❑ Milk Kefir	❑ Sunbathing	❑ Movement	❑ Ferments

Take a Moment:

If you find it in your heart to care for somebody else,
you will have succeeded. —Maya Angelou

Determine to care for someone else today. Write about what you did here.

_____

_____

_____

Today's Focus: _____

Nutritional Intake:

Breakfast _____

Mid-morning _____

Lunch _____

Mid-afternoon _____

Dinner _____

Evening _____

New Foods/Reactions: _____

Stools (amount, number and type): _____

Quick Symptoms Checklist: Rate Symptoms 0-10

❑ Headache	❑ Digestive symptoms	Energy level:_____
❑ Joint pain	❑ Abdominal pain	Mood: _____
❑ Muscle pain	❑ Tinnitus	Mental Clarity: _____
❑ Other: _____	❑ Other: _____	Purpose/Hope: _____

Date _____

❏ FCLO/HVBO	❏ Probiotic	❏ Detox Bath	❏ AM Juicing	❏ Fat
❏ Omega 3/6	❏ Beet Kvass	❏ Oil Pull	❏ PM Juicing	❏ Stock
❏ Iodine	❏ Milk Kefir	❏ Sunbathing	❏ Movement	❏ Ferments

Take a Moment:

Believe you can and you're halfway there. —Theodore Roosevelt

What do you need to believe today?

_____

_____

_____

_____

Today's Focus: _____

Nutritional Intake:

Breakfast _____

Mid-morning_____

Lunch _____

Mid-afternoon _____

Dinner _____

Evening _____

New Foods/Reactions: _____

Stools (amount, number and type): _____

Quick Symptoms Checklist: **Rate Symptoms 0-10**

❏ Headache	❏ Digestive symptoms	Energy level:_____
❏ Joint pain	❏ Abdominal pain	Mood: _____
❏ Muscle pain	❏ Tinnitus	Mental Clarity: _____
❏ Other: _____	❏ Other: _____	Purpose/Hope: _____

Date _____

❑ FCLO/HVBO	❑ Probiotic	❑ Detox Bath	❑ AM Juicing	❑ Fat
❑ Omega 3/6	❑ Beet Kvass	❑ Oil Pull	❑ PM Juicing	❑ Stock
❑ Iodine	❑ Milk Kefir	❑ Sunbathing	❑ Movement	❑ Ferments

Take a Moment:

> *The possession of knowledge does not kill the sense of wonder and mystery. There is always more mystery.* —Anaïs Nin

What is something that has recently caused you a feeling of wonder or mystery?

_____

_____

_____

Today's Focus: _____

Nutritional Intake:

Breakfast _____

Mid-morning _____

Lunch _____

Mid-afternoon _____

Dinner _____

Evening _____

New Foods/Reactions: _____

Stools (amount, number and type): _____

Quick Symptoms Checklist: **Rate Symptoms 0-10**

❑ Headache	❑ Digestive symptoms	Energy level:_____
❑ Joint pain	❑ Abdominal pain	Mood: _____
❑ Muscle pain	❑ Tinnitus	Mental Clarity: _____
❑ Other: _____	❑ Other: _____	Purpose/Hope: _____

Date _____

❏ FCLO/HVBO	❏ Probiotic	❏ Detox Bath	❏ AM Juicing	❏ Fat
❏ Omega 3/6	❏ Beet Kvass	❏ Oil Pull	❏ PM Juicing	❏ Stock
❏ Iodine	❏ Milk Kefir	❏ Sunbathing	❏ Movement	❏ Ferments

Take a Moment:

I couldn't wait for success, so I went ahead without it. —Jonathan Winters

Are you discouraged about your lack of success? How can you go ahead without it?

_____

_____

_____

Today's Focus: _____

Nutritional Intake:

Breakfast _____

Mid-morning_____

Lunch _____

Mid-afternoon _____

Dinner _____

Evening _____

New Foods/Reactions: _____

Stools (amount, number and type): _____

_____

Quick Symptoms Checklist: **Rate Symptoms 0-10**

❏ Headache	❏ Digestive symptoms	Energy level:_____
❏ Joint pain	❏ Abdominal pain	Mood: _____
❏ Muscle pain	❏ Tinnitus	Mental Clarity: _____
❏ Other: _____	❏ Other: _____	Purpose/Hope: _____

Date _____

❑ FCLO/HVBO	❑ Probiotic	❑ Detox Bath	❑ AM Juicing	❑ Fat
❑ Omega 3/6	❑ Beet Kvass	❑ Oil Pull	❑ PM Juicing	❑ Stock
❑ Iodine	❑ Milk Kefir	❑ Sunbathing	❑ Movement	❑ Ferments

Nutritional Intake:

Breakfast _____

Mid-morning _____

Lunch _____

Mid-afternoon _____

Dinner _____

Evening _____

New Foods/Reactions: _____

Stools (amount, number and type): _____

_____

Quick Symptoms Checklist: **Rate Symptoms 0-10**

❑ Headache	❑ Digestive symptoms	Energy level:_____
❑ Joint pain	❑ Abdominal pain	Mood: _____
❑ Muscle pain	❑ Tinnitus	Mental Clarity: _____
❑ Other: _____	❑ Other: _____	Purpose/Hope: _____

Date _____

❏ FCLO/HVBO	❏ Probiotic	❏ Detox Bath	❏ AM Juicing	❏ Fat
❏ Omega 3/6	❏ Beet Kvass	❏ Oil Pull	❏ PM Juicing	❏ Stock
❏ Iodine	❏ Milk Kefir	❏ Sunbathing	❏ Movement	❏ Ferments

Take a Moment:

What happens when people open their hearts? They get better.
—Haruki Murakami

This takes courage. Do you believe it could be true?

_____

_____

_____

Today's Focus: _____

Nutritional Intake:

Breakfast _____

Mid-morning _____

Lunch _____

Mid-afternoon _____

Dinner _____

Evening _____

New Foods/Reactions: _____

Stools (amount, number and type): _____

_____

Quick Symptoms Checklist: **Rate Symptoms 0-10**

❏ Headache	❏ Digestive symptoms	Energy level:_____
❏ Joint pain	❏ Abdominal pain	Mood: _____
❏ Muscle pain	❏ Tinnitus	Mental Clarity: _____
❏ Other: _____	❏ Other: _____	Purpose/Hope: _____

My week overall: 0--10

I would describe my week (in one word) as: _____

Because? _____

General progress:

Advanced to a new stage? Y/N   Current stage?_____

New foods tolerated: _____   Foods removed: _____

Animal fats consumed: _____   Avg. daily amount: _____

# of days stock consumed: _____   Avg. daily amount: _____

Probiotics/fermented foods/cultured dairy:

Probiotic supplement: _____Current dose: _____

Die-off symptoms: Y/N   Describe: _____

_____

Beet Kvass _____   Sour Cream _____

Veggie Medley_____   Yogurt _____

Sauerkraut_____   Kefir_____

Detoxing Progress:

# of detox baths: _____ Ingredients: ACV/Epsom/Baking soda

# of days sunbathed: _____ # of minutes per session:_____ minutes

# of days juiced in am: _____in pm: _____

Ingredients:_____

Overall reactions to detoxing: _____

Symptoms descriptions:

Stools: Daily Y/N   #per day _____   Type(s):_____

Digestion: _____

Mood/energy: _____

Memory/clarity: _____

Sleep/Stress: _____

Typical-for-me symptoms: _____

_____

Date _____

❏ FCLO/HVBO	❏ Probiotic	❏ Detox Bath	❏ AM Juicing	❏ Fat
❏ Omega 3/6	❏ Beet Kvass	❏ Oil Pull	❏ PM Juicing	❏ Stock
❏ Iodine	❏ Milk Kefir	❏ Sunbathing	❏ Movement	❏ Ferments

Take a Moment:

Never doubt that a small group of thoughtful, committed citizens can change the world. Indeed, it is the only thing that ever has.
—Margaret Mead

Are you tired of going against the flow. Can you believe that there is hope for change?

_____

_____

Today's Focus: _____

Nutritional Intake:

Breakfast _____

Mid-morning_____

Lunch _____

Mid-afternoon _____

Dinner _____

Evening _____

New Foods/Reactions:_____

Stools (amount, number and type): _____

_____

Quick Symptoms Checklist: **Rate Symptoms 0-10**

❏ Headache	❏ Digestive symptoms	Energy level:_____
❏ Joint pain	❏ Abdominal pain	Mood: _____
❏ Muscle pain	❏ Tinnitus	Mental Clarity: _____
❏ Other: _____	❏ Other: _____	Purpose/Hope: _____

Date _____

❏ FCLO/HVBO	❏ Probiotic	❏ Detox Bath	❏ AM Juicing	❏ Fat
❏ Omega 3/6	❏ Beet Kvass	❏ Oil Pull	❏ PM Juicing	❏ Stock
❏ Iodine	❏ Milk Kefir	❏ Sunbathing	❏ Movement	❏ Ferments

Take a Moment:

If you're going to be able to look back on something and laugh about it, you might as well laugh about it now. —Marie Osmond

Is there something you can laugh about now?

_____

_____

_____

Today's Focus: _____

Nutritional Intake:

Breakfast _____

Mid-morning _____

Lunch _____

Mid-afternoon _____

Dinner _____

Evening _____

New Foods/Reactions: _____

Stools (amount, number and type): _____

Quick Symptoms Checklist: Rate Symptoms 0-10

❏ Headache	❏ Digestive symptoms	Energy level: _____
❏ Joint pain	❏ Abdominal pain	Mood: _____
❏ Muscle pain	❏ Tinnitus	Mental Clarity: _____
❏ Other: _____	❏ Other: _____	Purpose/Hope: _____

Date _____

❑ FCLO/HVBO	❑ Probiotic	❑ Detox Bath	❑ AM Juicing	❑ Fat
❑ Omega 3/6	❑ Beet Kvass	❑ Oil Pull	❑ PM Juicing	❑ Stock
❑ Iodine	❑ Milk Kefir	❑ Sunbathing	❑ Movement	❑ Ferments

Take a Moment:

Begin at once to live, and count each separate day as a separate life.
—Seneca

Can you begin fresh again today?

_____

_____

_____

Today's Focus: _____

Nutritional Intake:

Breakfast _____

Mid-morning _____

Lunch _____

Mid-afternoon _____

Dinner _____

Evening _____

New Foods/Reactions: _____

Stools (amount, number and type): _____

_____

Quick Symptoms Checklist: **Rate Symptoms 0-10**

❑ Headache	❑ Digestive symptoms	Energy level:_____
❑ Joint pain	❑ Abdominal pain	Mood: _____
❑ Muscle pain	❑ Tinnitus	Mental Clarity: _____
❑ Other: _____	❑ Other: _____	Purpose/Hope: _____

Date _____

❏ FCLO/HVBO	❏ Probiotic	❏ Detox Bath	❏ AM Juicing	❏ Fat
❏ Omega 3/6	❏ Beet Kvass	❏ Oil Pull	❏ PM Juicing	❏ Stock
❏ Iodine	❏ Milk Kefir	❏ Sunbathing	❏ Movement	❏ Ferments

Take a Moment:

Friendship is born at that moment when one person says to another, 'What! You too! I thought I was the only one.' —C. S. Lewis

Who became your friend in this way? Let them know today that you are thankful for them.

_____

_____

_____

Today's Focus: _____

Nutritional Intake:

Breakfast _____

Mid-morning _____

Lunch _____

Mid-afternoon _____

Dinner _____

Evening _____

New Foods/Reactions: _____

Stools (amount, number and type): _____

_____

Quick Symptoms Checklist: Rate Symptoms 0-10

❏ Headache	❏ Digestive symptoms	Energy level:_____
❏ Joint pain	❏ Abdominal pain	Mood: _____
❏ Muscle pain	❏ Tinnitus	Mental Clarity:_____
❏ Other: _____	❏ Other: _____	Purpose/Hope: _____

Date _____

❏ FCLO/HVBO	❏ Probiotic	❏ Detox Bath	❏ AM Juicing	❏ Fat
❏ Omega 3/6	❏ Beet Kvass	❏ Oil Pull	❏ PM Juicing	❏ Stock
❏ Iodine	❏ Milk Kefir	❏ Sunbathing	❏ Movement	❏ Ferments

Take a Moment:

To live is the rarest thing in the world. Most people exist, that is all.
—Oscar Wilde

What would keep you from living today?

_____

_____

_____

Today's Focus: _____

Nutritional Intake:

Breakfast _____

Mid-morning_____

Lunch _____

Mid-afternoon _____

Dinner _____

Evening _____

New Foods/Reactions: _____

Stools (amount, number and type): _____

Quick Symptoms Checklist: **Rate Symptoms 0-10**

❏ Headache	❏ Digestive symptoms	Energy level:_____
❏ Joint pain	❏ Abdominal pain	Mood: _____
❏ Muscle pain	❏ Tinnitus	Mental Clarity:_____
❏ Other: _____	❏ Other: _____	Purpose/Hope: ____

Date _____

- ❑ FCLO/HVBO
- ❑ Omega 3/6
- ❑ Iodine
- ❑ Probiotic
- ❑ Beet Kvass
- ❑ Milk Kefir
- ❑ Detox Bath
- ❑ Oil Pull
- ❑ Sunbathing
- ❑ AM Juicing
- ❑ PM Juicing
- ❑ Movement
- ❑ Fat
- ❑ Stock
- ❑ Ferments

Take a Moment:

When a friend is in trouble, don't annoy him by asking if there is anything you can do. Think up something approprate and do it. —E.W. Howe

Have you been blessed by someone doing something for you? What can you do today for someone you know?

_____

_____

_____

Today's Focus: _____

Nutritional Intake:

Breakfast _____

Mid-morning_____

Lunch _____

Mid-afternoon _____

Dinner _____

Evening _____

New Foods/Reactions:_____

Stools (amount, number and type): _____

Quick Symptoms Checklist: Rate Symptoms 0-10

❑ Headache	❑ Digestive symptoms	Energy level:_____
❑ Joint pain	❑ Abdominal pain	Mood: _____
❑ Muscle pain	❑ Tinnitus	Mental Clarity:_____
❑ Other: _____	❑ Other: _____	Purpose/Hope: _____

Date _____

- ❏ FCLO/HVBO
- ❏ Omega 3/6
- ❏ Iodine
- ❏ Probiotic
- ❏ Beet Kvass
- ❏ Milk Kefir
- ❏ Detox Bath
- ❏ Oil Pull
- ❏ Sunbathing
- ❏ AM Juicing
- ❏ PM Juicing
- ❏ Movement
- ❏ Fat
- ❏ Stock
- ❏ Ferments

Take a Moment:

Enjoy the little things, for one day you may look back and realize they were the big things. —Robert Brault

Spend time today enjoying the little things.

_____

_____

_____

Today's Focus: _____

Nutritional Intake:

Breakfast _____

Mid-morning _____

Lunch _____

Mid-afternoon _____

Dinner _____

Evening _____

New Foods/Reactions: _____

Stools (amount, number and type): _____

Quick Symptoms Checklist: **Rate Symptoms 0-10**

- ❏ Headache
- ❏ Joint pain
- ❏ Muscle pain
- ❏ Other: _____
- ❏ Digestive symptoms
- ❏ Abdominal pain
- ❏ Tinnitus
- ❏ Other: _____

Energy level: _____
Mood: _____
Mental Clarity: _____
Purpose/Hope: _____

My week overall: 0--**10**

I would describe my week (in one word) as: _____

Because? _____

General progress:

Advanced to a new stage? Y/N   Current stage?_____

New foods tolerated: _____   Foods removed: _____

Animal fats consumed:_____   Avg. daily amount: _____

# of days stock consumed: _____   Avg. daily amount: _____

Probiotics/fermented foods/cultured dairy:

Probiotic supplement: _____Current dose: _____

Die-off symptoms: Y/N   Describe: _____

_____

Beet Kvass_____   Sour Cream_____

Veggie Medley_____   Yogurt _____

Sauerkraut_____   Kefir_____

Detoxing Progress:

# of detox baths: _____ Ingredients: ACV/Epsom/Baking soda

# of days sunbathed: _____ # of minutes per session:_____ minutes

# of days juiced in am: _____in pm: _____

Ingredients:_____

Overall reactions to detoxing: _____

Symptoms descriptions:

Stools: Daily Y/N   #per day _____   Type(s):_____

Digestion: _____

Mood/energy: _____

Memory/clarity: _____

Sleep/Stress: _____

Typical-for-me symptoms: _____

_____

Date _____

❑ FCLO/HVBO	❑ Probiotic	❑ Detox Bath	❑ AM Juicing	❑ Fat
❑ Omega 3/6	❑ Beet Kvass	❑ Oil Pull	❑ PM Juicing	❑ Stock
❑ Iodine	❑ Milk Kefir	❑ Sunbathing	❑ Movement	❑ Ferments

Take a Moment:

There are only two options regarding commitment. You're either in or you're out. There's no such thing as life in-between. —Pat Riley

Are you in? Can you commit to be in this week?

_____

_____

_____

Today's Focus: _____

Nutritional Intake:

Breakfast _____

Mid-morning _____

Lunch _____

Mid-afternoon _____

Dinner _____

Evening _____

New Foods/Reactions: _____

Stools (amount, number and type): _____

Quick Symptoms Checklist: **Rate Symptoms 0-10**

❑ Headache	❑ Digestive symptoms	Energy level:_____
❑ Joint pain	❑ Abdominal pain	Mood: _____
❑ Muscle pain	❑ Tinnitus	Mental Clarity: _____
❑ Other: _____	❑ Other: _____	Purpose/Hope: _____

Date _____

❑ FCLO/HVBO	❑ Probiotic	❑ Detox Bath	❑ AM Juicing	❑ Fat
❑ Omega 3/6	❑ Beet Kvass	❑ Oil Pull	❑ PM Juicing	❑ Stock
❑ Iodine	❑ Milk Kefir	❑ Sunbathing	❑ Movement	❑ Ferments

Take a Moment:

Everything that irritates us about others can lead us to an understanding of ourselves. —Carl Gustav Jung

Think about something that irritates you. What do you think that shows you about yourself?

_____

_____

_____

Today's Focus: _____

Nutritional Intake:

Breakfast _____

Mid-morning _____

Lunch _____

Mid-afternoon _____

Dinner _____

Evening _____

New Foods/Reactions: _____

Stools (amount, number and type): _____

Quick Symptoms Checklist: **Rate Symptoms 0-10**

❑ Headache	❑ Digestive symptoms	Energy level:_____
❑ Joint pain	❑ Abdominal pain	Mood: _____
❑ Muscle pain	❑ Tinnitus	Mental Clarity: _____
❑ Other: _____	❑ Other: _____	Purpose/Hope: _____

Date _____

❏ FCLO/HVBO	❏ Probiotic	❏ Detox Bath	❏ AM Juicing	❏ Fat
❏ Omega 3/6	❏ Beet Kvass	❏ Oil Pull	❏ PM Juicing	❏ Stock
❏ Iodine	❏ Milk Kefir	❏ Sunbathing	❏ Movement	❏ Ferments

Take a Moment:

I refuse to join any club that would not have me as a member. —Groucho Marx

You are in control of how others make you feel. What is your perspective today?

_____

_____

_____

Today's Focus: _____

Nutritional Intake:

Breakfast _____

Mid-morning_____

Lunch _____

Mid-afternoon _____

Dinner _____

Evening _____

New Foods/Reactions: _____

Stools (amount, number and type): _____

Quick Symptoms Checklist: Rate Symptoms 0-10

❏ Headache	❏ Digestive symptoms	Energy level:_____
❏ Joint pain	❏ Abdominal pain	Mood: _____
❏ Muscle pain	❏ Tinnitus	Mental Clarity:_____
❏ Other: _____	❏ Other: _____	Purpose/Hope: _____

Date _____

❏ FCLO/HVBO	❏ Probiotic	❏ Detox Bath	❏ AM Juicing	❏ Fat
❏ Omega 3/6	❏ Beet Kvass	❏ Oil Pull	❏ PM Juicing	❏ Stock
❏ Iodine	❏ Milk Kefir	❏ Sunbathing	❏ Movement	❏ Ferments

Take a Moment:

It's faith that will take you through, and determination that will drive you. —Johnathan Anthony Burkett

Where can you find faith today?

_____

_____

_____

Today's Focus: _____

Nutritional Intake:

Breakfast _____

Mid-morning _____

Lunch _____

Mid-afternoon _____

Dinner _____

Evening _____

New Foods/Reactions: _____

Stools (amount, number and type): _____

Quick Symptoms Checklist: Rate Symptoms 0-10

❏ Headache	❏ Digestive symptoms	Energy level: _____
❏ Joint pain	❏ Abdominal pain	Mood: _____
❏ Muscle pain	❏ Tinnitus	Mental Clarity: _____
❏ Other: _____	❏ Other: _____	Purpose/Hope: _____

Date _____

❏ FCLO/HVBO	❏ Probiotic	❏ Detox Bath	❏ AM Juicing	❏ Fat
❏ Omega 3/6	❏ Beet Kvass	❏ Oil Pull	❏ PM Juicing	❏ Stock
❏ Iodine	❏ Milk Kefir	❏ Sunbathing	❏ Movement	❏ Ferments

Take a Moment:

The two most powerful warriors are patience and time. —Leo Tolstoy

Do you have these warriors by your side today?

_____

_____

_____

_____

Today's Focus: _____

Nutritional Intake:

Breakfast _____

Mid-morning_____

Lunch _____

Mid-afternoon _____

Dinner _____

Evening _____

New Foods/Reactions: _____

Stools (amount, number and type): _____

_____

Quick Symptoms Checklist: **Rate Symptoms 0-10**

❏ Headache	❏ Digestive symptoms	Energy level:_____
❏ Joint pain	❏ Abdominal pain	Mood: _____
❏ Muscle pain	❏ Tinnitus	Mental Clarity:_____
❏ Other: _____	❏ Other: _____	Purpose/Hope: _____

Date _____

❏ FCLO/HVBO	❏ Probiotic	❏ Detox Bath	❏ AM Juicing	❏ Fat
❏ Omega 3/6	❏ Beet Kvass	❏ Oil Pull	❏ PM Juicing	❏ Stock
❏ Iodine	❏ Milk Kefir	❏ Sunbathing	❏ Movement	❏ Ferments

Take a Moment:

A positive attitude may not solve all your problems, but it will annoy enough people to make it worth the effort. —Herm Albright

I hope this quote made you laugh! Do you have a humorous story about this from your own life?

_____

_____

_____

Today's Focus: _____

Nutritional Intake:

Breakfast _____

Mid-morning _____

Lunch _____

Mid-afternoon _____

Dinner _____

Evening _____

New Foods/Reactions: _____

Stools (amount, number and type): _____

Quick Symptoms Checklist: Rate Symptoms 0-10

❏ Headache	❏ Digestive symptoms	Energy level: _____
❏ Joint pain	❏ Abdominal pain	Mood: _____
❏ Muscle pain	❏ Tinnitus	Mental Clarity: _____
❏ Other: _____	❏ Other: _____	Purpose/Hope: _____

Date _____

❏ FCLO/HVBO	❏ Probiotic	❏ Detox Bath	❏ AM Juicing	❏ Fat
❏ Omega 3/6	❏ Beet Kvass	❏ Oil Pull	❏ PM Juicing	❏ Stock
❏ Iodine	❏ Milk Kefir	❏ Sunbathing	❏ Movement	❏ Ferments

Take a Moment:

Sometimes we must yield control to others and accept our vulnerability so we can be healed. —Kathy Magliato

Do you need to yield control in something?

_____

_____

_____

Today's Focus: _____

Nutritional Intake:

Breakfast _____

Mid-morning _____

Lunch _____

Mid-afternoon _____

Dinner _____

Evening _____

New Foods/Reactions: _____

Stools (amount, number and type): _____

_____

Quick Symptoms Checklist:		**Rate Symptoms 0-10**
❏ Headache	❏ Digestive symptoms	Energy level: _____
❏ Joint pain	❏ Abdominal pain	Mood: _____
❏ Muscle pain	❏ Tinnitus	Mental Clarity: _____
❏ Other: _____	❏ Other: _____	Purpose/Hope: _____

My week overall: 0--10

I would describe my week (in one word) as: _____

Because? _____

General progress:

Advanced to a new stage? Y/N   Current stage?_____

New foods tolerated: _____   Foods removed: _____

Animal fats consumed: _____   Avg. daily amount: _____

# of days stock consumed: _____   Avg. daily amount: _____

Probiotics/fermented foods/cultured dairy:

Probiotic supplement: _____Current dose: _____

Die-off symptoms: Y/N   Describe: _____

_____

Beet Kvass _____   Sour Cream _____

Veggie Medley_____   Yogurt _____

Sauerkraut_____   Kefir_____

Detoxing Progress:

# of detox baths: _____ Ingredients: ACV/Epsom/Baking soda

# of days sunbathed: _____ # of minutes per session:_____ minutes

# of days juiced in am: _____in pm: _____

Ingredients:_____

Overall reactions to detoxing: _____

Symptoms descriptions:

Stools: Daily Y/N   #per day _____   Type(s):_____

Digestion: _____

Mood/energy: _____

Memory/clarity: _____

Sleep/Stress: _____

Typical-for-me symptoms: _____

_____

Date _____

❏ FCLO/HVBO	❏ Probiotic	❏ Detox Bath	❏ AM Juicing	❏ Fat
❏ Omega 3/6	❏ Beet Kvass	❏ Oil Pull	❏ PM Juicing	❏ Stock
❏ Iodine	❏ Milk Kefir	❏ Sunbathing	❏ Movement	❏ Ferments

Take a Moment:

> *Now and then it's good to pause in our pursuit of happiness and just be happy.* —Guillaume Apollinaire

Today, stop and just be happy. Write your thoughts.

_____

_____

_____

Today's Focus: _____

Nutritional Intake:

Breakfast _____

Mid-morning _____

Lunch _____

Mid-afternoon _____

Dinner _____

Evening _____

New Foods/Reactions: _____

Stools (amount, number and type): _____

Quick Symptoms Checklist: **Rate Symptoms 0-10**

❏ Headache	❏ Digestive symptoms	Energy level: _____
❏ Joint pain	❏ Abdominal pain	Mood: _____
❏ Muscle pain	❏ Tinnitus	Mental Clarity: _____
❏ Other: _____	❏ Other: _____	Purpose/Hope: _____

Date _____

❑ FCLO/HVBO	❑ Probiotic	❑ Detox Bath	❑ AM Juicing	❑ Fat
❑ Omega 3/6	❑ Beet Kvass	❑ Oil Pull	❑ PM Juicing	❑ Stock
❑ Iodine	❑ Milk Kefir	❑ Sunbathing	❑ Movement	❑ Ferments

Take a Moment:

> *I'm thankful for every moment.* —Al Green

Can you say this? Why or why not?

_____

_____

_____

_____

Today's Focus: _____

Nutritional Intake:

Breakfast _____

Mid-morning _____

Lunch _____

Mid-afternoon _____

Dinner _____

Evening _____

New Foods/Reactions: _____

Stools (amount, number and type): _____

_____

Quick Symptoms Checklist: **Rate Symptoms 0-10**

❑ Headache	❑ Digestive symptoms	Energy level:_____
❑ Joint pain	❑ Abdominal pain	Mood: _____
❑ Muscle pain	❑ Tinnitus	Mental Clarity: _____
❑ Other: _____	❑ Other: _____	Purpose/Hope: _____

Date _____

❏ FCLO/HVBO	❏ Probiotic	❏ Detox Bath	❏ AM Juicing	❏ Fat
❏ Omega 3/6	❏ Beet Kvass	❏ Oil Pull	❏ PM Juicing	❏ Stock
❏ Iodine	❏ Milk Kefir	❏ Sunbathing	❏ Movement	❏ Ferments

Take a Moment:

Most folks are about as happy as they make up their minds to be.
—Abraham Lincoln

How happy are you going to be today?

_____

_____

_____

Today's Focus: _____

Nutritional Intake:

Breakfast _____

Mid-morning_____

Lunch _____

Mid-afternoon _____

Dinner _____

Evening _____

New Foods/Reactions: _____

Stools (amount, number and type): _____

Quick Symptoms Checklist: **Rate Symptoms 0-10**

❏ Headache	❏ Digestive symptoms	Energy level:_____
❏ Joint pain	❏ Abdominal pain	Mood: _____
❏ Muscle pain	❏ Tinnitus	Mental Clarity: _____
❏ Other: _____	❏ Other: _____	Purpose/Hope: _____

Date _____

❑ FCLO/HVBO	❑ Probiotic	❑ Detox Bath	❑ AM Juicing	❑ Fat
❑ Omega 3/6	❑ Beet Kvass	❑ Oil Pull	❑ PM Juicing	❑ Stock
❑ Iodine	❑ Milk Kefir	❑ Sunbathing	❑ Movement	❑ Ferments

Take a Moment:

Do not take life to seriously. You will never get out alive. —Elbert Hubbard

Can you laugh a little today?

_____

_____

_____

_____

Today's Focus: _____

Nutritional Intake:

Breakfast _____

Mid-morning _____

Lunch _____

Mid-afternoon _____

Dinner _____

Evening _____

New Foods/Reactions: _____

Stools (amount, number and type): _____

Quick Symptoms Checklist: Rate Symptoms 0-10

❑ Headache	❑ Digestive symptoms	Energy level:_____
❑ Joint pain	❑ Abdominal pain	Mood: _____
❑ Muscle pain	❑ Tinnitus	Mental Clarity:_____
❑ Other: _____	❑ Other: _____	Purpose/Hope: _____

245

Date _____

❏ FCLO/HVBO	❏ Probiotic	❏ Detox Bath	❏ AM Juicing	❏ Fat
❏ Omega 3/6	❏ Beet Kvass	❏ Oil Pull	❏ PM Juicing	❏ Stock
❏ Iodine	❏ Milk Kefir	❏ Sunbathing	❏ Movement	❏ Ferments

Take a Moment:

To enjoy freedom we have to control ourselves. —Virginia Woolf

What do you think about this? Does this seem like freedom?

_____

_____

_____

_____

Today's Focus: _____

Nutritional Intake:

Breakfast _____

Mid-morning _____

Lunch _____

Mid-afternoon _____

Dinner _____

Evening _____

New Foods/Reactions: _____

Stools (amount, number and type): _____

_____

Quick Symptoms Checklist: **Rate Symptoms 0-10**

❏ Headache	❏ Digestive symptoms	Energy level:_____
❏ Joint pain	❏ Abdominal pain	Mood: _____
❏ Muscle pain	❏ Tinnitus	Mental Clarity: _____
❏ Other: _____	❏ Other: _____	Purpose/Hope: _____

Date _____

❏ FCLO/HVBO	❏ Probiotic	❏ Detox Bath	❏ AM Juicing	❏ Fat
❏ Omega 3/6	❏ Beet Kvass	❏ Oil Pull	❏ PM Juicing	❏ Stock
❏ Iodine	❏ Milk Kefir	❏ Sunbathing	❏ Movement	❏ Ferments

Take a Moment:

> *Even the smallest shift in perspective can bring about the greatest healing.* —Joshua Kai

Have you experienced this before? Share it here.

_____

_____

_____

Today's Focus: _____

Nutritional Intake:

Breakfast _____

Mid-morning _____

Lunch _____

Mid-afternoon _____

Dinner _____

Evening _____

New Foods/Reactions: _____

Stools (amount, number and type): _____

_____

Quick Symptoms Checklist: Rate Symptoms 0-10

❏ Headache	❏ Digestive symptoms	Energy level:_____
❏ Joint pain	❏ Abdominal pain	Mood: _____
❏ Muscle pain	❏ Tinnitus	Mental Clarity: _____
❏ Other: _____	❏ Other: _____	Purpose/Hope: _____

Date _____

❏ FCLO/HVBO	❏ Probiotic	❏ Detox Bath	❏ AM Juicing	❏ Fat
❏ Omega 3/6	❏ Beet Kvass	❏ Oil Pull	❏ PM Juicing	❏ Stock
❏ Iodine	❏ Milk Kefir	❏ Sunbathing	❏ Movement	❏ Ferments

Take a Moment:

I try to forget what happiness was, and when that don't work,
I study the stars. —Derek Walcott

Stargaze. If you want, write your thoughts.

_____

_____

_____

Today's Focus: _____

Nutritional Intake:

Breakfast _____

Mid-morning_____

Lunch _____

Mid-afternoon _____

Dinner _____

Evening _____

New Foods/Reactions: _____

Stools (amount, number and type): _____

Quick Symptoms Checklist: **Rate Symptoms 0-10**

❏ Headache	❏ Digestive symptoms	Energy level:_____
❏ Joint pain	❏ Abdominal pain	Mood: _____
❏ Muscle pain	❏ Tinnitus	Mental Clarity: _____
❏ Other: _____	❏ Other: _____	Purpose/Hope: _____

My week overall: 0--10

I would describe my week (in one word) as: _____

Because? _____

General progress:

Advanced to a new stage? Y/N   Current stage?_____

New foods tolerated: _____   Foods removed: _____

Animal fats consumed: _____   Avg. daily amount: _____

# of days stock consumed: _____   Avg. daily amount: _____

Probiotics/fermented foods/cultured dairy:

Probiotic supplement: _____Current dose: _____

Die-off symptoms: Y/N   Describe: _____

_____

Beet Kvass _____   Sour Cream _____

Veggie Medley_____   Yogurt _____

Sauerkraut_____   Kefir_____

Detoxing Progress:

# of detox baths: _____ Ingredients: ACV/Epsom/Baking soda

# of days sunbathed: _____ # of minutes per session:_____ minutes

# of days juiced in am: _____in pm: _____

Ingredients:_____

Overall reactions to detoxing: _____

Symptoms descriptions:

Stools: Daily Y/N   #per day _____   Type(s):_____

Digestion: _____

Mood/energy: _____

Memory/clarity: _____

Sleep/Stress: _____

Typical-for-me symptoms: _____

_____

Date _____

❑ FCLO/HVBO	❑ Probiotic	❑ Detox Bath	❑ AM Juicing	❑ Fat
❑ Omega 3/6	❑ Beet Kvass	❑ Oil Pull	❑ PM Juicing	❑ Stock
❑ Iodine	❑ Milk Kefir	❑ Sunbathing	❑ Movement	❑ Ferments

Take a Moment:

Don't find the time to exercise, make the time to exercise. —Unknown

Exercise to your current level of health, but exercise! Make a plan to exercise next week.

_____

_____

_____

Today's Focus: _____

Nutritional Intake:

Breakfast _____

Mid-morning_____

Lunch _____

Mid-afternoon _____

Dinner _____

Evening _____

New Foods/Reactions: _____

Stools (amount, number and type): _____

Quick Symptoms Checklist:		Rate Symptoms 0-10
❑ Headache	❑ Digestive symptoms	Energy level:_____
❑ Joint pain	❑ Abdominal pain	Mood: _____
❑ Muscle pain	❑ Tinnitus	Mental Clarity:_____
❑ Other: _____	❑ Other: _____	Purpose/Hope: _____

Date _____

❑ FCLO/HVBO	❑ Probiotic	❑ Detox Bath	❑ AM Juicing	❑ Fat
❑ Omega 3/6	❑ Beet Kvass	❑ Oil Pull	❑ PM Juicing	❑ Stock
❑ Iodine	❑ Milk Kefir	❑ Sunbathing	❑ Movement	❑ Ferments

Take a Moment:

Cutting out bad habits is far more effective than cutting out organs.
—Herbert M. Shelton

Is there a bad habit you need to cut out, starting today?

_____

_____

_____

Today's Focus: _____

Nutritional Intake:

Breakfast _____

Mid-morning _____

Lunch _____

Mid-afternoon _____

Dinner _____

Evening _____

New Foods/Reactions: _____

Stools (amount, number and type): _____

_____

Quick Symptoms Checklist: **Rate Symptoms 0-10**

❑ Headache	❑ Digestive symptoms	Energy level:_____
❑ Joint pain	❑ Abdominal pain	Mood: _____
❑ Muscle pain	❑ Tinnitus	Mental Clarity: _____
❑ Other: _____	❑ Other: _____	Purpose/Hope: _____

Date _____

❏ FCLO/HVBO	❏ Probiotic	❏ Detox Bath	❏ AM Juicing	❏ Fat
❏ Omega 3/6	❏ Beet Kvass	❏ Oil Pull	❏ PM Juicing	❏ Stock
❏ Iodine	❏ Milk Kefir	❏ Sunbathing	❏ Movement	❏ Ferments

Take a Moment:

The race is not always to the swift, but to those who keep on running.
—Anonymous

What keeps you motivated to keep running?

_____

_____

_____

Today's Focus: _____

Nutritional Intake:

Breakfast _____

Mid-morning_____

Lunch _____

Mid-afternoon _____

Dinner _____

Evening _____

New Foods/Reactions: _____

Stools (amount, number and type): _____

_____

Quick Symptoms Checklist: **Rate Symptoms 0-10**

❏ Headache	❏ Digestive symptoms	Energy level:_____
❏ Joint pain	❏ Abdominal pain	Mood: _____
❏ Muscle pain	❏ Tinnitus	Mental Clarity: _____
❏ Other: _____	❏ Other: _____	Purpose/Hope: _____

Date _____

❏ FCLO/HVBO	❏ Probiotic	❏ Detox Bath	❏ AM Juicing	❏ Fat
❏ Omega 3/6	❏ Beet Kvass	❏ Oil Pull	❏ PM Juicing	❏ Stock
❏ Iodine	❏ Milk Kefir	❏ Sunbathing	❏ Movement	❏ Ferments

Take a Moment:

All generalizations are false, including this one. —Mark Twain

A little humor and truth for today. Have you generalized anything recently that you shouldn't have?

_____

_____

_____

Today's Focus: _____

Nutritional Intake:

Breakfast _____

Mid-morning _____

Lunch _____

Mid-afternoon _____

Dinner _____

Evening _____

New Foods/Reactions: _____

Stools (amount, number and type): _____

_____

Quick Symptoms Checklist: Rate Symptoms 0-10

❏ Headache	❏ Digestive symptoms	Energy level: _____
❏ Joint pain	❏ Abdominal pain	Mood: _____
❏ Muscle pain	❏ Tinnitus	Mental Clarity: _____
❏ Other: _____	❏ Other: _____	Purpose/Hope: _____

Date _____

❏ FCLO/HVBO	❏ Probiotic	❏ Detox Bath	❏ AM Juicing	❏ Fat
❏ Omega 3/6	❏ Beet Kvass	❏ Oil Pull	❏ PM Juicing	❏ Stock
❏ Iodine	❏ Milk Kefir	❏ Sunbathing	❏ Movement	❏ Ferments

Take a Moment:

My theory is to enjoy life, but the practice is against it . —Andrew Sachs

It can be hard to enjoy life . . . how are you successful?

_____

_____

_____

_____

Today's Focus: _____

Nutritional Intake:

Breakfast _____

Mid-morning_____

Lunch _____

Mid-afternoon _____

Dinner _____

Evening _____

New Foods/Reactions: _____

Stools (amount, number and type): _____

_____

Quick Symptoms Checklist:		**Rate Symptoms 0-10**
❏ Headache	❏ Digestive symptoms	Energy level:_____
❏ Joint pain	❏ Abdominal pain	Mood: _____
❏ Muscle pain	❏ Tinnitus	Mental Clarity: _____
❏ Other: _____	❏ Other: _____	Purpose/Hope: _____

Date _____

❏ FCLO/HVBO	❏ Probiotic	❏ Detox Bath	❏ AM Juicing	❏ Fat
❏ Omega 3/6	❏ Beet Kvass	❏ Oil Pull	❏ PM Juicing	❏ Stock
❏ Iodine	❏ Milk Kefir	❏ Sunbathing	❏ Movement	❏ Ferments

Take a Moment:

... stories that rise from deep suffering can provide the most potent remedies for past, present and even future ills. —Clarissa Pinkola Estés

Do you have a story? Share it if you want.

_____

_____

_____

Today's Focus: _____

Nutritional Intake:

Breakfast _____

Mid-morning _____

Lunch _____

Mid-afternoon _____

Dinner _____

Evening _____

New Foods/Reactions: _____

Stools (amount, number and type): _____

_____

Quick Symptoms Checklist: **Rate Symptoms 0-10**

❏ Headache	❏ Digestive symptoms	Energy level: _____
❏ Joint pain	❏ Abdominal pain	Mood: _____
❏ Muscle pain	❏ Tinnitus	Mental Clarity: _____
❏ Other: _____	❏ Other: _____	Purpose/Hope: _____

Date _____

❏ FCLO/HVBO	❏ Probiotic	❏ Detox Bath	❏ AM Juicing	❏ Fat
❏ Omega 3/6	❏ Beet Kvass	❏ Oil Pull	❏ PM Juicing	❏ Stock
❏ Iodine	❏ Milk Kefir	❏ Sunbathing	❏ Movement	❏ Ferments

Take a Moment:

Rest is not idleness, and to lie sometimes on the grass under trees on a summer's day, listening to the murmur of the water, or watching the clouds float across the sky, is by no means a waste of time. —John Lubbock

Spend some time resting today.

_____

_____

_____

Today's Focus: _____

Nutritional Intake:

Breakfast _____

Mid-morning _____

Lunch _____

Mid-afternoon _____

Dinner _____

Evening _____

New Foods/Reactions: _____

Stools (amount, number and type): _____

_____

Quick Symptoms Checklist:		**Rate Symptoms 0-10**
❏ Headache	❏ Digestive symptoms	Energy level:_____
❏ Joint pain	❏ Abdominal pain	Mood: _____
❏ Muscle pain	❏ Tinnitus	Mental Clarity: _____
❏ Other: _____	❏ Other: _____	Purpose/Hope: _____

Week-At-A-Glance

My week overall: 0--**10**

I would describe my week (in one word) as: _____

Because? _____

General progress:

Advanced to a new stage? Y/N   Current stage?_____

New foods tolerated: _____   Foods removed: _____

Animal fats consumed: _____   Avg. daily amount: _____

# of days stock consumed: _____   Avg. daily amount: _____

Probiotics/fermented foods/cultured dairy:

Probiotic supplement: _____Current dose: _____

Die-off symptoms: Y/N   Describe: _____

_____

Beet Kvass_____   Sour Cream_____

Veggie Medley_____   Yogurt _____

Sauerkraut_____   Kefir_____

Detoxing Progress:

# of detox baths: _____ Ingredients: ACV/Epsom/Baking soda

# of days sunbathed: _____ # of minutes per session:_____ minutes

# of days juiced in am: _____in pm: _____

Ingredients:_____

Overall reactions to detoxing: _____

Symptoms descriptions:

Stools: Daily Y/N   #per day _____   Type(s):_____

Digestion: _____

Mood/energy: _____

Memory/clarity: _____

Sleep/Stress: _____

Typical-for-me symptoms: _____

_____

Date _____

❑ FCLO/HVBO	❑ Probiotic	❑ Detox Bath	❑ AM Juicing	❑ Fat
❑ Omega 3/6	❑ Beet Kvass	❑ Oil Pull	❑ PM Juicing	❑ Stock
❑ Iodine	❑ Milk Kefir	❑ Sunbathing	❑ Movement	❑ Ferments

Take a Moment:

Isn't it nice to think that tomorrow is a new day with no mistakes in it yet? —L.M. Montgomery

Are you excited for a new day tomorrow?

_____

_____

_____

Today's Focus: _____

Nutritional Intake:

Breakfast _____

Mid-morning _____

Lunch _____

Mid-afternoon _____

Dinner _____

Evening _____

New Foods/Reactions: _____

Stools (amount, number and type): _____

_____

Quick Symptoms Checklist:		**Rate Symptoms 0-10**
❑ Headache	❑ Digestive symptoms	Energy level:_____
❑ Joint pain	❑ Abdominal pain	Mood: _____
❑ Muscle pain	❑ Tinnitus	Mental Clarity:_____
❑ Other: _____	❑ Other: _____	Purpose/Hope:_____

Date _____

❑ FCLO/HVBO	❑ Probiotic	❑ Detox Bath	❑ AM Juicing	❑ Fat
❑ Omega 3/6	❑ Beet Kvass	❑ Oil Pull	❑ PM Juicing	❑ Stock
❑ Iodine	❑ Milk Kefir	❑ Sunbathing	❑ Movement	❑ Ferments

Take a Moment:

If you don't take care of the most magnificent machine that you will ever be given . . . where are you going to live? —Karyn Calabrese

Do you find it hard to take time to care for your body?

_____

_____

_____

Today's Focus: _____

Nutritional Intake:

Breakfast _____

Mid-morning_____

Lunch _____

Mid-afternoon _____

Dinner _____

Evening _____

New Foods/Reactions: _____

Stools (amount, number and type): _____

_____

Quick Symptoms Checklist: Rate Symptoms 0-10

❑ Headache	❑ Digestive symptoms	Energy level:_____
❑ Joint pain	❑ Abdominal pain	Mood: _____
❑ Muscle pain	❑ Tinnitus	Mental Clarity: _____
❑ Other: _____	❑ Other: _____	Purpose/Hope: _____

Date _____

❑ FCLO/HVBO	❑ Probiotic	❑ Detox Bath	❑ AM Juicing	❑ Fat
❑ Omega 3/6	❑ Beet Kvass	❑ Oil Pull	❑ PM Juicing	❑ Stock
❑ Iodine	❑ Milk Kefir	❑ Sunbathing	❑ Movement	❑ Ferments

Take a Moment:

When you make a choice, you change the future. —Deepak Chopra

What is a choice that you will make today?

_____

_____

_____

Today's Focus: _____

Nutritional Intake:

Breakfast _____

Mid-morning_____

Lunch _____

Mid-afternoon _____

Dinner _____

Evening _____

New Foods/Reactions:_____

Stools (amount, number and type): _____

_____

Quick Symptoms Checklist: **Rate Symptoms 0-10**

❑ Headache	❑ Digestive symptoms	Energy level:_____
❑ Joint pain	❑ Abdominal pain	Mood: _____
❑ Muscle pain	❑ Tinnitus	Mental Clarity: _____
❑ Other: _____	❑ Other: _____	Purpose/Hope: _____

Date _____

❏ FCLO/HVBO	❏ Probiotic	❏ Detox Bath	❏ AM Juicing	❏ Fat
❏ Omega 3/6	❏ Beet Kvass	❏ Oil Pull	❏ PM Juicing	❏ Stock
❏ Iodine	❏ Milk Kefir	❏ Sunbathing	❏ Movement	❏ Ferments

Take a Moment:

It's not whether you get knocked down, it's whether you get back up.
—Vince Lombardi

Do you feel knocked down? How can you get up again?

_____

_____

_____

Today's Focus: _____

Nutritional Intake:

Breakfast _____

Mid-morning _____

Lunch _____

Mid-afternoon _____

Dinner _____

Evening _____

New Foods/Reactions: _____

Stools (amount, number and type): _____

_____

Quick Symptoms Checklist: **Rate Symptoms 0-10**

❏ Headache	❏ Digestive symptoms	Energy level: _____
❏ Joint pain	❏ Abdominal pain	Mood: _____
❏ Muscle pain	❏ Tinnitus	Mental Clarity: _____
❏ Other: _____	❏ Other: _____	Purpose/Hope: _____

Date _____

❏ FCLO/HVBO	❏ Probiotic	❏ Detox Bath	❏ AM Juicing	❏ Fat
❏ Omega 3/6	❏ Beet Kvass	❏ Oil Pull	❏ PM Juicing	❏ Stock
❏ Iodine	❏ Milk Kefir	❏ Sunbathing	❏ Movement	❏ Ferments

Take a Moment:

> *Appreciation is a wonderful thing. It makes what is excellent in others belong to us as well.* —Voltair

What do you appreciate about someone? Tell them today.

_____

_____

_____

Today's Focus: _____

Nutritional Intake:

Breakfast _____

Mid-morning _____

Lunch _____

Mid-afternoon _____

Dinner _____

Evening _____

New Foods/Reactions: _____

Stools (amount, number and type): _____

_____

Quick Symptoms Checklist:		Rate Symptoms 0-10
❏ Headache	❏ Digestive symptoms	Energy level:_____
❏ Joint pain	❏ Abdominal pain	Mood: _____
❏ Muscle pain	❏ Tinnitus	Mental Clarity: _____
❏ Other: _____	❏ Other: _____	Purpose/Hope: _____

Date _____

❏ FCLO/HVBO	❏ Probiotic	❏ Detox Bath	❏ AM Juicing	❏ Fat
❏ Omega 3/6	❏ Beet Kvass	❏ Oil Pull	❏ PM Juicing	❏ Stock
❏ Iodine	❏ Milk Kefir	❏ Sunbathing	❏ Movement	❏ Ferments

Take a Moment:

Letting ourselves be forgiven is one of the most difficult healings we will undertake. And one of the most fruitful. —Stephen Levine

What is something that you are not allowing yourself be forgiven in?

_____

_____

_____

Today's Focus: _____

Nutritional Intake:

Breakfast _____

Mid-morning _____

Lunch _____

Mid-afternoon _____

Dinner _____

Evening _____

New Foods/Reactions: _____

Stools (amount, number and type): _____

_____

Quick Symptoms Checklist: Rate Symptoms 0-10

❏ Headache	❏ Digestive symptoms	Energy level:_____
❏ Joint pain	❏ Abdominal pain	Mood: _____
❏ Muscle pain	❏ Tinnitus	Mental Clarity: _____
❏ Other: _____	❏ Other: _____	Purpose/Hope: _____

Date _____

❏ FCLO/HVBO	❏ Probiotic	❏ Detox Bath	❏ AM Juicing	❏ Fat
❏ Omega 3/6	❏ Beet Kvass	❏ Oil Pull	❏ PM Juicing	❏ Stock
❏ Iodine	❏ Milk Kefir	❏ Sunbathing	❏ Movement	❏ Ferments

Take a Moment:

Moderation. Small helpings. Sample a little bit of everything. These are the secrets of happiness and good health. —Julia Child

At this time you probably shouldn't taste every food. But what foods that you can eat should you maybe take in more moderation?

_____
_____
_____

Today's Focus: _____

Nutritional Intake:

Breakfast _____

Mid-morning _____

Lunch _____

Mid-afternoon _____

Dinner _____

Evening _____

New Foods/Reactions: _____

Stools (amount, number and type): _____

Quick Symptoms Checklist: **Rate Symptoms 0-10**

❏ Headache	❏ Digestive symptoms	Energy level:_____
❏ Joint pain	❏ Abdominal pain	Mood: _____
❏ Muscle pain	❏ Tinnitus	Mental Clarity: _____
❏ Other: _____	❏ Other: _____	Purpose/Hope: _____

My week overall: 0--**10**

I would describe my week (in one word) as: _____

Because? _____

General progress:

Advanced to a new stage? Y/N   Current stage?_____

New foods tolerated: _____   Foods removed: _____

Animal fats consumed: _____   Avg. daily amount: _____

# of days stock consumed: _____   Avg. daily amount: _____

Probiotics/fermented foods/cultured dairy:

Probiotic supplement: _____Current dose: _____

Die-off symptoms: Y/N   Describe: _____

_____

Beet Kvass _____   Sour Cream _____

Veggie Medley _____   Yogurt _____

Sauerkraut_____   Kefir_____

Detoxing Progress:

# of detox baths: _____ Ingredients: ACV/Epsom/Baking soda

# of days sunbathed: _____ # of minutes per session:_____ minutes

# of days juiced in am: _____in pm: _____

Ingredients:_____

Overall reactions to detoxing: _____

Symptoms descriptions:

Stools: Daily Y/N   #per day _____   Type(s):_____

Digestion: _____

Mood/energy: _____

Memory/clarity: _____

Sleep/Stress: _____

Typical-for-me symptoms: _____

_____

Date _____

❏ FCLO/HVBO	❏ Probiotic	❏ Detox Bath	❏ AM Juicing	❏ Fat
❏ Omega 3/6	❏ Beet Kvass	❏ Oil Pull	❏ PM Juicing	❏ Stock
❏ Iodine	❏ Milk Kefir	❏ Sunbathing	❏ Movement	❏ Ferments

Take a Moment:

> *What drains your spirit drains your body. What fuels your spirit fuels your body.* —Caroline Myss

Do something that fuels your spirit (and body) today.

_____

_____

_____

Today's Focus: _____

Nutritional Intake:

Breakfast _____

Mid-morning _____

Lunch _____

Mid-afternoon _____

Dinner _____

Evening _____

New Foods/Reactions: _____

Stools (amount, number and type): _____

Quick Symptoms Checklist: **Rate Symptoms 0-10**

❏ Headache	❏ Digestive symptoms	Energy level:_____
❏ Joint pain	❏ Abdominal pain	Mood: _____
❏ Muscle pain	❏ Tinnitus	Mental Clarity: _____
❏ Other: _____	❏ Other: _____	Purpose/Hope: _____

Date _____

❏ FCLO/HVBO	❏ Probiotic	❏ Detox Bath	❏ AM Juicing	❏ Fat
❏ Omega 3/6	❏ Beet Kvass	❏ Oil Pull	❏ PM Juicing	❏ Stock
❏ Iodine	❏ Milk Kefir	❏ Sunbathing	❏ Movement	❏ Ferments

Take a Moment:

Caring about the hapiness of others, we find our own. —Plato

Who can you care about today?

_____

_____

_____

_____

Today's Focus: _____

Nutritional Intake:

Breakfast _____

Mid-morning _____

Lunch _____

Mid-afternoon _____

Dinner _____

Evening _____

New Foods/Reactions: _____

Stools (amount, number and type): _____

Quick Symptoms Checklist: **Rate Symptoms 0-10**

❏ Headache	❏ Digestive symptoms	Energy level:_____
❏ Joint pain	❏ Abdominal pain	Mood: _____
❏ Muscle pain	❏ Tinnitus	Mental Clarity: _____
❏ Other: _____	❏ Other: _____	Purpose/Hope: ____

Date _____

❏ FCLO/HVBO	❏ Probiotic	❏ Detox Bath	❏ AM Juicing	❏ Fat
❏ Omega 3/6	❏ Beet Kvass	❏ Oil Pull	❏ PM Juicing	❏ Stock
❏ Iodine	❏ Milk Kefir	❏ Sunbathing	❏ Movement	❏ Ferments

Take a Moment:

> *No person was ever honored for what he received. Honor has been the reward for what he gave.* —Calvin Coolidge

What can you give today?

_____

_____

_____

Today's Focus: _____

Nutritional Intake:

Breakfast _____

Mid-morning_____

Lunch _____

Mid-afternoon _____

Dinner _____

Evening _____

New Foods/Reactions: _____

Stools (amount, number and type): _____

Quick Symptoms Checklist: **Rate Symptoms 0-10**

❏ Headache	❏ Digestive symptoms	Energy level:_____
❏ Joint pain	❏ Abdominal pain	Mood: _____
❏ Muscle pain	❏ Tinnitus	Mental Clarity: _____
❏ Other: _____	❏ Other: _____	Purpose/Hope: _____

Date _____

❑ FCLO/HVBO	❑ Probiotic	❑ Detox Bath	❑ AM Juicing	❑ Fat
❑ Omega 3/6	❑ Beet Kvass	❑ Oil Pull	❑ PM Juicing	❑ Stock
❑ Iodine	❑ Milk Kefir	❑ Sunbathing	❑ Movement	❑ Ferments

Take a Moment:

Every morning is a beautiful morning. —Terri Guillemets

Why is this morning beautiful?

_____

_____

_____

Today's Focus: _____

Nutritional Intake:

Breakfast _____

Mid-morning_____

Lunch _____

Mid-afternoon _____

Dinner _____

Evening _____

New Foods/Reactions: _____

Stools (amount, number and type): _____

_____

Quick Symptoms Checklist: Rate Symptoms 0-10

❑ Headache	❑ Digestive symptoms	Energy level:_____
❑ Joint pain	❑ Abdominal pain	Mood: _____
❑ Muscle pain	❑ Tinnitus	Mental Clarity:_____
❑ Other: _____	❑ Other: _____	Purpose/Hope: _____

Date _____

❑ FCLO/HVBO	❑ Probiotic	❑ Detox Bath	❑ AM Juicing	❑ Fat
❑ Omega 3/6	❑ Beet Kvass	❑ Oil Pull	❑ PM Juicing	❑ Stock
❑ Iodine	❑ Milk Kefir	❑ Sunbathing	❑ Movement	❑ Ferments

Take a Moment:

> *Do what you can, with what you have, with where you are.*
> —Theodore Roosevelt

What can you do with what you have today?

_____

_____

_____

Today's Focus: _____

Nutritional Intake:

Breakfast _____

Mid-morning_____

Lunch _____

Mid-afternoon _____

Dinner _____

Evening _____

New Foods/Reactions: _____

Stools (amount, number and type): _____

_____

Quick Symptoms Checklist:		**Rate Symptoms 0-10**
❑ Headache	❑ Digestive symptoms	Energy level:_____
❑ Joint pain	❑ Abdominal pain	Mood: _____
❑ Muscle pain	❑ Tinnitus	Mental Clarity: _____
❑ Other: _____	❑ Other: _____	Purpose/Hope: _____

Date _____

❑ FCLO/HVBO	❑ Probiotic	❑ Detox Bath	❑ AM Juicing	❑ Fat
❑ Omega 3/6	❑ Beet Kvass	❑ Oil Pull	❑ PM Juicing	❑ Stock
❑ Iodine	❑ Milk Kefir	❑ Sunbathing	❑ Movement	❑ Ferments

Take a Moment:

I will not say: do not weep; for not all tears are an evil. —J.R.R. Tolkien

When have tears, even sad tears, been good?

_____

_____

_____

_____

Today's Focus: _____

Nutritional Intake:

Breakfast _____

Mid-morning _____

Lunch _____

Mid-afternoon _____

Dinner _____

Evening _____

New Foods/Reactions: _____

Stools (amount, number and type): _____

_____

Quick Symptoms Checklist: Rate Symptoms 0-10

❑ Headache	❑ Digestive symptoms	Energy level:_____
❑ Joint pain	❑ Abdominal pain	Mood: _____
❑ Muscle pain	❑ Tinnitus	Mental Clarity: _____
❑ Other: _____	❑ Other: _____	Purpose/Hope: _____

Date _____

❑ FCLO/HVBO	❑ Probiotic	❑ Detox Bath	❑ AM Juicing	❑ Fat
❑ Omega 3/6	❑ Beet Kvass	❑ Oil Pull	❑ PM Juicing	❑ Stock
❑ Iodine	❑ Milk Kefir	❑ Sunbathing	❑ Movement	❑ Ferments

Take a Moment:

To weep is to make less the depth of grief. —William Shakespeare

Spend time crying today, if you can.

_____

_____

_____

_____

Today's Focus: _____

Nutritional Intake:

Breakfast _____

Mid-morning_____

Lunch _____

Mid-afternoon _____

Dinner _____

Evening _____

New Foods/Reactions: _____

Stools (amount, number and type): _____

_____

Quick Symptoms Checklist: **Rate Symptoms 0-10**

❑ Headache	❑ Digestive symptoms	Energy level:_____
❑ Joint pain	❑ Abdominal pain	Mood: _____
❑ Muscle pain	❑ Tinnitus	Mental Clarity: _____
❑ Other: _____	❑ Other: _____	Purpose/Hope: _____

My week overall: 0---**10**

I would describe my week (in one word) as: _____

Because? _____

General progress:

Advanced to a new stage? Y/N   Current stage?_____

New foods tolerated: _____   Foods removed: _____

Animal fats consumed: _____   Avg. daily amount: _____

# of days stock consumed: _____   Avg. daily amount: _____

Probiotics/fermented foods/cultured dairy:

Probiotic supplement: _____Current dose: _____

Die-off symptoms: Y/N   Describe: _____

_____

Beet Kvass _____   Sour Cream _____

Veggie Medley_____   Yogurt _____

Sauerkraut_____   Kefir_____

Detoxing Progress:

# of detox baths: _____ Ingredients: ACV/Epsom/Baking soda

# of days sunbathed: _____ # of minutes per session:_____ minutes

# of days juiced in am: _____in pm: _____

Ingredients:_____

Overall reactions to detoxing: _____

Symptoms descriptions:

Stools: Daily Y/N   #per day _____   Type(s):_____

Digestion: _____

Mood/energy: _____

Memory/clarity: _____

Sleep/Stress: _____

Typical-for-me symptoms: _____

_____

Date _____

❑ FCLO/HVBO	❑ Probiotic	❑ Detox Bath	❑ AM Juicing	❑ Fat
❑ Omega 3/6	❑ Beet Kvass	❑ Oil Pull	❑ PM Juicing	❑ Stock
❑ Iodine	❑ Milk Kefir	❑ Sunbathing	❑ Movement	❑ Ferments

Take a Moment:

Even if I knew that tomorrow the world would go to pieces, I would still plant my apple tree. —Martin Luther

It takes a calm spirit to hope for tomorrow when things seem uncertain. What gives you hope today?

_____

_____

_____

Today's Focus: _____

Nutritional Intake:

Breakfast _____

Mid-morning_____

Lunch _____

Mid-afternoon _____

Dinner _____

Evening _____

New Foods/Reactions:_____

Stools (amount, number and type): _____

_____

Quick Symptoms Checklist: **Rate Symptoms 0-10**

❑ Headache	❑ Digestive symptoms	Energy level:_____
❑ Joint pain	❑ Abdominal pain	Mood: _____
❑ Muscle pain	❑ Tinnitus	Mental Clarity: _____
❑ Other: _____	❑ Other: _____	Purpose/Hope: _____

Date _____

❑ FCLO/HVBO	❑ Probiotic	❑ Detox Bath	❑ AM Juicing	❑ Fat
❑ Omega 3/6	❑ Beet Kvass	❑ Oil Pull	❑ PM Juicing	❑ Stock
❑ Iodine	❑ Milk Kefir	❑ Sunbathing	❑ Movement	❑ Ferments

Take a Moment:

Stop seeking out the storms and enjoy more fully the sunlight.
—Gordon B. Hinckley

Plenty of storms come, but sometimes we look for them.
How can you enjoy the sunlight today?

_____

_____

_____

Today's Focus: _____

Nutritional Intake:

Breakfast _____

Mid-morning _____

Lunch _____

Mid-afternoon _____

Dinner _____

Evening _____

New Foods/Reactions: _____

Stools (amount, number and type): _____

Quick Symptoms Checklist: Rate Symptoms 0-10

❑ Headache	❑ Digestive symptoms	Energy level:_____
❑ Joint pain	❑ Abdominal pain	Mood: _____
❑ Muscle pain	❑ Tinnitus	Mental Clarity: _____
❑ Other: _____	❑ Other: _____	Purpose/Hope: _____

Date _____

❏ FCLO/HVBO	❏ Probiotic	❏ Detox Bath	❏ AM Juicing	❏ Fat
❏ Omega 3/6	❏ Beet Kvass	❏ Oil Pull	❏ PM Juicing	❏ Stock
❏ Iodine	❏ Milk Kefir	❏ Sunbathing	❏ Movement	❏ Ferments

Take a Moment:

Some wounds were worth bearing for the healing they brought.
—Dianna Hardy

What healing have you gotten from a worthwhile wound.

_____

_____

_____

Today's Focus: _____

Nutritional Intake:

Breakfast _____

Mid-morning_____

Lunch _____

Mid-afternoon _____

Dinner _____

Evening _____

New Foods/Reactions: _____

Stools (amount, number and type): _____

Quick Symptoms Checklist: **Rate Symptoms 0-10**

❏ Headache	❏ Digestive symptoms	Energy level:_____
❏ Joint pain	❏ Abdominal pain	Mood: _____
❏ Muscle pain	❏ Tinnitus	Mental Clarity: _____
❏ Other: _____	❏ Other: _____	Purpose/Hope: _____

Date _____

❏ FCLO/HVBO	❏ Probiotic	❏ Detox Bath	❏ AM Juicing	❏ Fat
❏ Omega 3/6	❏ Beet Kvass	❏ Oil Pull	❏ PM Juicing	❏ Stock
❏ Iodine	❏ Milk Kefir	❏ Sunbathing	❏ Movement	❏ Ferments

Take a Moment:

To strengthen the muscles of your heart, the best exercise is lifting someone else's spirit whenever you can. —Dodinsky

Who's spirit can you lift today? Write about it.

_____

_____

_____

Today's Focus: _____

Nutritional Intake:

Breakfast _____

Mid-morning _____

Lunch _____

Mid-afternoon _____

Dinner _____

Evening _____

New Foods/Reactions: _____

Stools (amount, number and type): _____

Quick Symptoms Checklist: Rate Symptoms 0-10

❏ Headache	❏ Digestive symptoms	Energy level:_____
❏ Joint pain	❏ Abdominal pain	Mood: _____
❏ Muscle pain	❏ Tinnitus	Mental Clarity: _____
❏ Other: _____	❏ Other: _____	Purpose/Hope: _____

Date _____

❏ FCLO/HVBO	❏ Probiotic	❏ Detox Bath	❏ AM Juicing	❏ Fat
❏ Omega 3/6	❏ Beet Kvass	❏ Oil Pull	❏ PM Juicing	❏ Stock
❏ Iodine	❏ Milk Kefir	❏ Sunbathing	❏ Movement	❏ Ferments

Take a Moment:

> *Keep your eyes open to your mercies. The man who forgets to be thankful has fallen asleep in life.* —Robert Louis Stevenson

Don't forget to be thankful. What are you thankful for today?"

_____

_____

_____

Today's Focus: _____

Nutritional Intake:

Breakfast _____

Mid-morning_____

Lunch _____

Mid-afternoon _____

Dinner _____

Evening _____

New Foods/Reactions: _____

Stools (amount, number and type): _____

Quick Symptoms Checklist: **Rate Symptoms 0-10**

❏ Headache	❏ Digestive symptoms	Energy level:_____
❏ Joint pain	❏ Abdominal pain	Mood: _____
❏ Muscle pain	❏ Tinnitus	Mental Clarity: _____
❏ Other: _____	❏ Other: _____	Purpose/Hope: _____

Date _____

❑ FCLO/HVBO	❑ Probiotic	❑ Detox Bath	❑ AM Juicing	❑ Fat
❑ Omega 3/6	❑ Beet Kvass	❑ Oil Pull	❑ PM Juicing	❑ Stock
❑ Iodine	❑ Milk Kefir	❑ Sunbathing	❑ Movement	❑ Ferments

Take a Moment:

Instead of saying, 'I'm damaged, I'm broken, I have trust issues'
say 'I'm healing, I'm rediscovering myself, I'm starting over.
—Horacio Jones

Self talk is loud. Replace some of your negative self talk today!

_____

_____

_____

Today's Focus: _____

Nutritional Intake:

Breakfast _____

Mid-morning_____

Lunch _____

Mid-afternoon _____

Dinner _____

Evening _____

New Foods/Reactions: _____

Stools (amount, number and type): _____

_____

Quick Symptoms Checklist: Rate Symptoms 0-10

❑ Headache	❑ Digestive symptoms	Energy level:_____
❑ Joint pain	❑ Abdominal pain	Mood: _____
❑ Muscle pain	❑ Tinnitus	Mental Clarity: _____
❑ Other: _____	❑ Other: _____	Purpose/Hope: _____

Date _____

❑ FCLO/HVBO	❑ Probiotic	❑ Detox Bath	❑ AM Juicing	❑ Fat
❑ Omega 3/6	❑ Beet Kvass	❑ Oil Pull	❑ PM Juicing	❑ Stock
❑ Iodine	❑ Milk Kefir	❑ Sunbathing	❑ Movement	❑ Ferments

Take a Moment:

When we face the worst that can happen in any situation, we grow.
When circumstances are at their worst, we can find our best.
—Elisabeth Kübler-Ross

Is something making you grow right now?

_____

_____

_____

Today's Focus: _____

Nutritional Intake:

Breakfast _____

Mid-morning_____

Lunch _____

Mid-afternoon _____

Dinner _____

Evening _____

New Foods/Reactions:_____

Stools (amount, number and type): _____

_____

Quick Symptoms Checklist: **Rate Symptoms 0-10**

❑ Headache	❑ Digestive symptoms	Energy level:_____
❑ Joint pain	❑ Abdominal pain	Mood: _____
❑ Muscle pain	❑ Tinnitus	Mental Clarity: _____
❑ Other: _____	❑ Other: _____	Purpose/Hope: _____

Week-At-A-Glance

My week overall: 0--10

I would describe my week (in one word) as: _____

Because? _____

General progress:

Advanced to a new stage? Y/N   Current stage?_____

New foods tolerated: _____   Foods removed: _____

Animal fats consumed: _____   Avg. daily amount: _____

# of days stock consumed: _____   Avg. daily amount: _____

Probiotics/fermented foods/cultured dairy:

Probiotic supplement: _____Current dose: _____

Die-off symptoms: Y/N   Describe: _____

_____

Beet Kvass _____   Sour Cream _____

Veggie Medley_____   Yogurt _____

Sauerkraut_____   Kefir_____

Detoxing Progress:

# of detox baths: _____ Ingredients: ACV/Epsom/Baking soda

# of days sunbathed: _____ # of minutes per session:_____ minutes

# of days juiced in am: _____in pm: _____

Ingredients:_____

Overall reactions to detoxing: _____

Symptoms descriptions:

Stools: Daily Y/N   #per day _____   Type(s):_____

Digestion: _____

Mood/energy: _____

Memory/clarity: _____

Sleep/Stress: _____

Typical-for-me symptoms: _____

_____

Date _____

❏ FCLO/HVBO	❏ Probiotic	❏ Detox Bath	❏ AM Juicing	❏ Fat
❏ Omega 3/6	❏ Beet Kvass	❏ Oil Pull	❏ PM Juicing	❏ Stock
❏ Iodine	❏ Milk Kefir	❏ Sunbathing	❏ Movement	❏ Ferments

Take a Moment:

Nature uses human imagination to lift her work of creation to even higher levels. —Luigi Pirandello

Take time today looking at the clouds and letting your imagination go.

_____

_____

_____

Today's Focus: _____

Nutritional Intake:

Breakfast _____

Mid-morning _____

Lunch _____

Mid-afternoon _____

Dinner _____

Evening _____

New Foods/Reactions: _____

Stools (amount, number and type): _____

Quick Symptoms Checklist: **Rate Symptoms 0-10**

❏ Headache	❏ Digestive symptoms	Energy level:_____
❏ Joint pain	❏ Abdominal pain	Mood: _____
❏ Muscle pain	❏ Tinnitus	Mental Clarity: _____
❏ Other: _____	❏ Other: _____	Purpose/Hope: _____

Date _____

❏ FCLO/HVBO	❏ Probiotic	❏ Detox Bath	❏ AM Juicing	❏ Fat
❏ Omega 3/6	❏ Beet Kvass	❏ Oil Pull	❏ PM Juicing	❏ Stock
❏ Iodine	❏ Milk Kefir	❏ Sunbathing	❏ Movement	❏ Ferments

Take a Moment:

Always Do Your Best. Your best is going to change from moment to moment; it will be different when you are healthy as opposed to sick. Under any circumstance, simply do your best, and you will avoid self-judgement, self-abuse and regret. —Don Miguel Ruiz

Are you happy with yourself when you do your best for that moment?

_____

_____

Today's Focus: _____

Nutritional Intake:

Breakfast _____

Mid-morning _____

Lunch _____

Mid-afternoon _____

Dinner _____

Evening _____

New Foods/Reactions: _____

Stools (amount, number and type): _____

Quick Symptoms Checklist: Rate Symptoms 0-10

❏ Headache	❏ Digestive symptoms	Energy level:_____
❏ Joint pain	❏ Abdominal pain	Mood: _____
❏ Muscle pain	❏ Tinnitus	Mental Clarity:_____
❏ Other: _____	❏ Other: _____	Purpose/Hope:_____

Date _____

❏ FCLO/HVBO	❏ Probiotic	❏ Detox Bath	❏ AM Juicing	❏ Fat
❏ Omega 3/6	❏ Beet Kvass	❏ Oil Pull	❏ PM Juicing	❏ Stock
❏ Iodine	❏ Milk Kefir	❏ Sunbathing	❏ Movement	❏ Ferments

Take a Moment:

Each day is filled with promise, potential and possibility. —Tony Curl

What do you think is today's potential?

_____

_____

_____

_____

Today's Focus: _____

Nutritional Intake:

Breakfast _____

Mid-morning _____

Lunch _____

Mid-afternoon _____

Dinner _____

Evening _____

New Foods/Reactions: _____

Stools (amount, number and type): _____

_____

Quick Symptoms Checklist: **Rate Symptoms 0-10**

❏ Headache	❏ Digestive symptoms	Energy level:_____
❏ Joint pain	❏ Abdominal pain	Mood: _____
❏ Muscle pain	❏ Tinnitus	Mental Clarity:_____
❏ Other: _____	❏ Other: _____	Purpose/Hope: ____

Date _____

❏ FCLO/HVBO	❏ Probiotic	❏ Detox Bath	❏ AM Juicing	❏ Fat
❏ Omega 3/6	❏ Beet Kvass	❏ Oil Pull	❏ PM Juicing	❏ Stock
❏ Iodine	❏ Milk Kefir	❏ Sunbathing	❏ Movement	❏ Ferments

Take a Moment:

Humor does not diminish the pain—it makes the space around it get bigger. —Allen Klein

Do you need a little space today?

_____

_____

_____

Today's Focus: _____

Nutritional Intake:

Breakfast _____

Mid-morning _____

Lunch _____

Mid-afternoon _____

Dinner _____

Evening _____

New Foods/Reactions: _____

Stools (amount, number and type): _____

_____

Quick Symptoms Checklist: Rate Symptoms 0-10

❏ Headache	❏ Digestive symptoms	Energy level:_____
❏ Joint pain	❏ Abdominal pain	Mood: _____
❏ Muscle pain	❏ Tinnitus	Mental Clarity: _____
❏ Other: _____	❏ Other: _____	Purpose/Hope: _____

Date _____

❑ FCLO/HVBO	❑ Probiotic	❑ Detox Bath	❑ AM Juicing	❑ Fat
❑ Omega 3/6	❑ Beet Kvass	❑ Oil Pull	❑ PM Juicing	❑ Stock
❑ Iodine	❑ Milk Kefir	❑ Sunbathing	❑ Movement	❑ Ferments

Take a Moment:

> *There is no illness that is not exacerbated by stress.* —Alan Lokos

Is stress affecting you today? Can you reduce it in any way?

_____

_____

_____

_____

Today's Focus: _____

Nutritional Intake:

Breakfast _____

Mid-morning _____

Lunch _____

Mid-afternoon _____

Dinner _____

Evening _____

New Foods/Reactions: _____

Stools (amount, number and type): _____

Quick Symptoms Checklist: **Rate Symptoms 0-10**

❑ Headache	❑ Digestive symptoms	Energy level:_____
❑ Joint pain	❑ Abdominal pain	Mood: _____
❑ Muscle pain	❑ Tinnitus	Mental Clarity: _____
❑ Other: _____	❑ Other: _____	Purpose/Hope: _____

Date _____

❏ FCLO/HVBO ❏ Probiotic ❏ Detox Bath ❏ AM Juicing ❏ Fat
❏ Omega 3/6 ❏ Beet Kvass ❏ Oil Pull ❏ PM Juicing ❏ Stock
❏ Iodine ❏ Milk Kefir ❏ Sunbathing ❏ Movement ❏ Ferments

Take a Moment:

Joy is a decision, a really brave one, about how you are going to respond to life. —Wess Stafford

Write about a time that you chose joy.

_____

_____

_____

Today's Focus: _____

Nutritional Intake:

Breakfast _____

Mid-morning _____

Lunch _____

Mid-afternoon _____

Dinner _____

Evening _____

New Foods/Reactions: _____

Stools (amount, number and type): _____

Quick Symptoms Checklist: Rate Symptoms 0-10

❏ Headache ❏ Digestive symptoms Energy level: _____
❏ Joint pain ❏ Abdominal pain Mood: _____
❏ Muscle pain ❏ Tinnitus Mental Clarity: _____
❏ Other: _____ ❏ Other: _____ Purpose/Hope: _____

Date _____

❏ FCLO/HVBO	❏ Probiotic	❏ Detox Bath	❏ AM Juicing	❏ Fat
❏ Omega 3/6	❏ Beet Kvass	❏ Oil Pull	❏ PM Juicing	❏ Stock
❏ Iodine	❏ Milk Kefir	❏ Sunbathing	❏ Movement	❏ Ferments

Take a Moment:

Character cannot be developed in ease and quiet. Only through experience of trial and suffering can the soul be strengthened, ambition inspired, and success achieved. —Helen Keller

What has trial and suffering produced in you?

_____

_____

_____

Today's Focus: _____

Nutritional Intake:

Breakfast _____

Mid-morning_____

Lunch _____

Mid-afternoon _____

Dinner _____

Evening _____

New Foods/Reactions:_____

Stools (amount, number and type): _____

Quick Symptoms Checklist: **Rate Symptoms 0-10**

❏ Headache	❏ Digestive symptoms	Energy level:_____
❏ Joint pain	❏ Abdominal pain	Mood: _____
❏ Muscle pain	❏ Tinnitus	Mental Clarity: _____
❏ Other: _____	❏ Other: _____	Purpose/Hope: _____

My week overall: 0---10

I would describe my week (in one word) as: _____

Because? _____

General progress:

Advanced to a new stage? Y/N   Current stage?_____

New foods tolerated: _____   Foods removed: _____

Animal fats consumed: _____   Avg. daily amount: _____

# of days stock consumed: _____   Avg. daily amount: _____

Probiotics/fermented foods/cultured dairy:

Probiotic supplement: _____Current dose: _____

Die-off symptoms: Y/N   Describe: _____

_____

Beet Kvass _____   Sour Cream _____

Veggie Medley _____   Yogurt _____

Sauerkraut_____   Kefir_____

Detoxing Progress:

# of detox baths: _____ Ingredients: ACV/Epsom/Baking soda

# of days sunbathed: _____ # of minutes per session:_____ minutes

# of days juiced in am: _____in pm: _____

Ingredients:_____

Overall reactions to detoxing: _____

Symptoms descriptions:

Stools: Daily Y/N   #per day _____   Type(s):_____

Digestion: _____

Mood/energy: _____

Memory/clarity: _____

Sleep/Stress: _____

Typical-for-me symptoms: _____

_____

Date _____

❏ FCLO/HVBO	❏ Probiotic	❏ Detox Bath	❏ AM Juicing	❏ Fat
❏ Omega 3/6	❏ Beet Kvass	❏ Oil Pull	❏ PM Juicing	❏ Stock
❏ Iodine	❏ Milk Kefir	❏ Sunbathing	❏ Movement	❏ Ferments

Take a Moment:

I think the next best thing to solving a problem is finding some humor in it. —Frank A. Clark

Are you facing an unsolvable problem? Can you find some humor in it?

_____

_____

_____

Today's Focus: _____

Nutritional Intake:

Breakfast _____

Mid-morning_____

Lunch _____

Mid-afternoon _____

Dinner _____

Evening _____

New Foods/Reactions:_____

Stools (amount, number and type): _____

_____

Quick Symptoms Checklist:		**Rate Symptoms 0-10**
❏ Headache	❏ Digestive symptoms	Energy level:_____
❏ Joint pain	❏ Abdominal pain	Mood: _____
❏ Muscle pain	❏ Tinnitus	Mental Clarity:_____
❏ Other: _____	❏ Other: _____	Purpose/Hope: _____

Date _____

❏ FCLO/HVBO	❏ Probiotic	❏ Detox Bath	❏ AM Juicing	❏ Fat
❏ Omega 3/6	❏ Beet Kvass	❏ Oil Pull	❏ PM Juicing	❏ Stock
❏ Iodine	❏ Milk Kefir	❏ Sunbathing	❏ Movement	❏ Ferments

Take a Moment:

A kind gesture can reach a wound that only compassion can heal.
—Steve Maraboli

Do something kind today. You have no idea what wound it may heal.

_____

_____

_____

Today's Focus: _____

Nutritional Intake:

Breakfast _____

Mid-morning _____

Lunch _____

Mid-afternoon _____

Dinner _____

Evening _____

New Foods/Reactions: _____

Stools (amount, number and type): _____

Quick Symptoms Checklist: Rate Symptoms 0-10

❏ Headache	❏ Digestive symptoms	Energy level: _____
❏ Joint pain	❏ Abdominal pain	Mood: _____
❏ Muscle pain	❏ Tinnitus	Mental Clarity: _____
❏ Other: _____	❏ Other: _____	Purpose/Hope: _____

Date _____

❏ FCLO/HVBO	❏ Probiotic	❏ Detox Bath	❏ AM Juicing	❏ Fat
❏ Omega 3/6	❏ Beet Kvass	❏ Oil Pull	❏ PM Juicing	❏ Stock
❏ Iodine	❏ Milk Kefir	❏ Sunbathing	❏ Movement	❏ Ferments

Take a Moment:

A happy person is not without sorrow or grief. Happiness is the acceptance of pain, not the lack of it. —Vironika Tugaleva

What do you think about this? Does it seem true to you?

_____

_____

_____

Today's Focus: _____

Nutritional Intake:

Breakfast _____

Mid-morning_____

Lunch _____

Mid-afternoon _____

Dinner _____

Evening _____

New Foods/Reactions: _____

Stools (amount, number and type): _____

Quick Symptoms Checklist: **Rate Symptoms 0-10**

❏ Headache	❏ Digestive symptoms	Energy level:_____
❏ Joint pain	❏ Abdominal pain	Mood: _____
❏ Muscle pain	❏ Tinnitus	Mental Clarity: _____
❏ Other: _____	❏ Other: _____	Purpose/Hope: _____

Date _____

❑ FCLO/HVBO	❑ Probiotic	❑ Detox Bath	❑ AM Juicing	❑ Fat
❑ Omega 3/6	❑ Beet Kvass	❑ Oil Pull	❑ PM Juicing	❑ Stock
❑ Iodine	❑ Milk Kefir	❑ Sunbathing	❑ Movement	❑ Ferments

Take a Moment:

Let us be grateful to people who make us happy; they are the charming gardeners who make our souls blossom. —Marcel Proust

Who has helped your soul blossom? Thank them today.

_____

_____

_____

Today's Focus: _____

Nutritional Intake:

Breakfast _____

Mid-morning _____

Lunch _____

Mid-afternoon _____

Dinner _____

Evening _____

New Foods/Reactions: _____

Stools (amount, number and type): _____

Quick Symptoms Checklist: **Rate Symptoms 0-10**

❑ Headache	❑ Digestive symptoms	Energy level: _____
❑ Joint pain	❑ Abdominal pain	Mood: _____
❑ Muscle pain	❑ Tinnitus	Mental Clarity: _____
❑ Other: _____	❑ Other: _____	Purpose/Hope: _____

Date _____

❑ FCLO/HVBO	❑ Probiotic	❑ Detox Bath	❑ AM Juicing	❑ Fat
❑ Omega 3/6	❑ Beet Kvass	❑ Oil Pull	❑ PM Juicing	❑ Stock
❑ Iodine	❑ Milk Kefir	❑ Sunbathing	❑ Movement	❑ Ferments

Take a Moment:

Tomorrow is not a promise. Tomorrow is a second chance. —J.R. Rim

What are you glad you get a second chance to do today?

_____

_____

_____

_____

Today's Focus: _____

Nutritional Intake:

Breakfast _____

Mid-morning _____

Lunch _____

Mid-afternoon _____

Dinner _____

Evening _____

New Foods/Reactions: _____

Stools (amount, number and type): _____

_____

Quick Symptoms Checklist: Rate Symptoms 0-10

❑ Headache	❑ Digestive symptoms	Energy level: _____
❑ Joint pain	❑ Abdominal pain	Mood: _____
❑ Muscle pain	❑ Tinnitus	Mental Clarity: _____
❑ Other: _____	❑ Other: _____	Purpose/Hope: _____

Date _____

❑ FCLO/HVBO	❑ Probiotic	❑ Detox Bath	❑ AM Juicing	❑ Fat
❑ Omega 3/6	❑ Beet Kvass	❑ Oil Pull	❑ PM Juicing	❑ Stock
❑ Iodine	❑ Milk Kefir	❑ Sunbathing	❑ Movement	❑ Ferments

Take a Moment:

A certain amount of opposition is a great help to a man. Kites rise against, not with, the wind. —John Neal

How has opposition helped you to rise?

_____

_____

_____

Today's Focus: _____

Nutritional Intake:

Breakfast _____

Mid-morning _____

Lunch _____

Mid-afternoon _____

Dinner _____

Evening _____

New Foods/Reactions: _____

Stools (amount, number and type): _____

_____

Quick Symptoms Checklist: Rate Symptoms 0-10

❑ Headache	❑ Digestive symptoms	Energy level: _____
❑ Joint pain	❑ Abdominal pain	Mood: _____
❑ Muscle pain	❑ Tinnitus	Mental Clarity: _____
❑ Other: _____	❑ Other: _____	Purpose/Hope: _____

Date _____

❑ FCLO/HVBO	❑ Probiotic	❑ Detox Bath	❑ AM Juicing	❑ Fat
❑ Omega 3/6	❑ Beet Kvass	❑ Oil Pull	❑ PM Juicing	❑ Stock
❑ Iodine	❑ Milk Kefir	❑ Sunbathing	❑ Movement	❑ Ferments

Take a Moment:

Autumn is a second spring when every leaf is a flower. —Albert Camus

Take time to see the beauty in the outside world around you today.

_____

_____

_____

_____

Today's Focus: _____

Nutritional Intake:

Breakfast _____

Mid-morning _____

Lunch _____

Mid-afternoon _____

Dinner _____

Evening _____

New Foods/Reactions: _____

Stools (amount, number and type): _____

_____

Quick Symptoms Checklist: **Rate Symptoms 0-10**

❑ Headache	❑ Digestive symptoms	Energy level:_____
❑ Joint pain	❑ Abdominal pain	Mood: _____
❑ Muscle pain	❑ Tinnitus	Mental Clarity: _____
❑ Other: _____	❑ Other: _____	Purpose/Hope: _____

My week overall: 0--10

I would describe my week (in one word) as: _____

Because? _____

General progress:

Advanced to a new stage? Y/N   Current stage?_____

New foods tolerated: _____   Foods removed: _____

Animal fats consumed: _____   Avg. daily amount: _____

# of days stock consumed: _____   Avg. daily amount: _____

Probiotics/fermented foods/cultured dairy:

Probiotic supplement: _____Current dose: _____

Die-off symptoms: Y/N   Describe: _____

_____

Beet Kvass _____   Sour Cream _____

Veggie Medley_____   Yogurt _____

Sauerkraut_____   Kefir_____

Detoxing Progress:

# of detox baths: _____ Ingredients: ACV/Epsom/Baking soda

# of days sunbathed: _____ # of minutes per session:_____ minutes

# of days juiced in am: _____in pm: _____

Ingredients:_____

Overall reactions to detoxing: _____

Symptoms descriptions:

Stools: Daily Y/N   #per day _____   Type(s):_____

Digestion: _____

Mood/energy: _____

Memory/clarity: _____

Sleep/Stress: _____

Typical-for-me symptoms: _____

_____

Date _____

❑ FCLO/HVBO	❑ Probiotic	❑ Detox Bath	❑ AM Juicing	❑ Fat
❑ Omega 3/6	❑ Beet Kvass	❑ Oil Pull	❑ PM Juicing	❑ Stock
❑ Iodine	❑ Milk Kefir	❑ Sunbathing	❑ Movement	❑ Ferments

Take a Moment:

> *Although the world is full of suffering, it's full also of the overcoming it.* —Helen Keller

Do you feel like you can overcome what you are going through?

_____

_____

_____

Today's Focus: _____

Nutritional Intake:

Breakfast _____

Mid-morning _____

Lunch _____

Mid-afternoon _____

Dinner _____

Evening _____

New Foods/Reactions: _____

Stools (amount, number and type): _____

Quick Symptoms Checklist: **Rate Symptoms 0-10**

❑ Headache	❑ Digestive symptoms	Energy level:_____
❑ Joint pain	❑ Abdominal pain	Mood: _____
❑ Muscle pain	❑ Tinnitus	Mental Clarity:_____
❑ Other: _____	❑ Other: _____	Purpose/Hope: _____

Date _____

❑ FCLO/HVBO	❑ Probiotic	❑ Detox Bath	❑ AM Juicing	❑ Fat
❑ Omega 3/6	❑ Beet Kvass	❑ Oil Pull	❑ PM Juicing	❑ Stock
❑ Iodine	❑ Milk Kefir	❑ Sunbathing	❑ Movement	❑ Ferments

Take a Moment:

Expect to have hope rekindled. Expect your prayers to be answered in wondrous ways. The dry seasons do not last. The spring rains will come. —Sarah Ban Breathnach

Are you in a dry spell. Do you have any hope?

_____

_____

_____

Today's Focus: _____

Nutritional Intake:

Breakfast _____

Mid-morning_____

Lunch _____

Mid-afternoon _____

Dinner _____

Evening _____

New Foods/Reactions: _____

Stools (amount, number and type): _____

_____

Quick Symptoms Checklist: **Rate Symptoms 0-10**

❑ Headache	❑ Digestive symptoms	Energy level:_____
❑ Joint pain	❑ Abdominal pain	Mood: _____
❑ Muscle pain	❑ Tinnitus	Mental Clarity:_____
❑ Other: _____	❑ Other: _____	Purpose/Hope: _____

Date _____

❏ FCLO/HVBO	❏ Probiotic	❏ Detox Bath	❏ AM Juicing	❏ Fat
❏ Omega 3/6	❏ Beet Kvass	❏ Oil Pull	❏ PM Juicing	❏ Stock
❏ Iodine	❏ Milk Kefir	❏ Sunbathing	❏ Movement	❏ Ferments

Take a Moment:

> *Faith moves mountains. If faith were easy there would be no mountains.* —Immaculée Ilibagiza

Keeping faith is hard. Do you have any today?

_____

_____

_____

Today's Focus: _____

Nutritional Intake:

Breakfast _____

Mid-morning_____

Lunch _____

Mid-afternoon _____

Dinner _____

Evening _____

New Foods/Reactions: _____

Stools (amount, number and type): _____

Quick Symptoms Checklist: **Rate Symptoms 0-10**

❏ Headache	❏ Digestive symptoms	Energy level:_____
❏ Joint pain	❏ Abdominal pain	Mood: _____
❏ Muscle pain	❏ Tinnitus	Mental Clarity: _____
❏ Other: _____	❏ Other: _____	Purpose/Hope: _____

Date _____

❑ FCLO/HVBO	❑ Probiotic	❑ Detox Bath	❑ AM Juicing	❑ Fat
❑ Omega 3/6	❑ Beet Kvass	❑ Oil Pull	❑ PM Juicing	❑ Stock
❑ Iodine	❑ Milk Kefir	❑ Sunbathing	❑ Movement	❑ Ferments

Take a Moment:

The most wasted of all days is one without laughter. —E.E. Cummings

What can you laugh about today?

_____

_____

_____

_____

Today's Focus: _____

Nutritional Intake:

Breakfast _____

Mid-morning _____

Lunch _____

Mid-afternoon _____

Dinner _____

Evening _____

New Foods/Reactions: _____

Stools (amount, number and type): _____

Quick Symptoms Checklist: **Rate Symptoms 0-10**

❑ Headache	❑ Digestive symptoms	Energy level:_____
❑ Joint pain	❑ Abdominal pain	Mood: _____
❑ Muscle pain	❑ Tinnitus	Mental Clarity: _____
❑ Other: _____	❑ Other: _____	Purpose/Hope: _____

Date _____

❏ FCLO/HVBO	❏ Probiotic	❏ Detox Bath	❏ AM Juicing	❏ Fat
❏ Omega 3/6	❏ Beet Kvass	❏ Oil Pull	❏ PM Juicing	❏ Stock
❏ Iodine	❏ Milk Kefir	❏ Sunbathing	❏ Movement	❏ Ferments

Take a Moment:

Be a good listener . . . It makes the person who's speaking to you feel loved, cared for and worthy of being heard. —Wayne Dyer

Today, instead of talking, listen to somone else. Write about it here.

_____

_____

_____

Today's Focus: _____

Nutritional Intake:

Breakfast _____

Mid-morning _____

Lunch _____

Mid-afternoon _____

Dinner _____

Evening _____

New Foods/Reactions: _____

Stools (amount, number and type): _____

Quick Symptoms Checklist: **Rate Symptoms 0-10**

❏ Headache	❏ Digestive symptoms	Energy level: _____
❏ Joint pain	❏ Abdominal pain	Mood: _____
❏ Muscle pain	❏ Tinnitus	Mental Clarity: _____
❏ Other: _____	❏ Other: _____	Purpose/Hope: _____

Date _____

❑ FCLO/HVBO	❑ Probiotic	❑ Detox Bath	❑ AM Juicing	❑ Fat
❑ Omega 3/6	❑ Beet Kvass	❑ Oil Pull	❑ PM Juicing	❑ Stock
❑ Iodine	❑ Milk Kefir	❑ Sunbathing	❑ Movement	❑ Ferments

Take a Moment:

With every mistake, we must surely be learning. —George Harrison

What have you learned from a recent mistake?

_____

_____

_____

_____

Today's Focus: _____

Nutritional Intake:

Breakfast _____

Mid-morning _____

Lunch _____

Mid-afternoon _____

Dinner _____

Evening _____

New Foods/Reactions: _____

Stools (amount, number and type): _____

Quick Symptoms Checklist: **Rate Symptoms 0-10**

❑ Headache	❑ Digestive symptoms	Energy level:_____
❑ Joint pain	❑ Abdominal pain	Mood: _____
❑ Muscle pain	❑ Tinnitus	Mental Clarity:_____
❑ Other: _____	❑ Other: _____	Purpose/Hope: _____

Date _____

❑ FCLO/HVBO	❑ Probiotic	❑ Detox Bath	❑ AM Juicing	❑ Fat
❑ Omega 3/6	❑ Beet Kvass	❑ Oil Pull	❑ PM Juicing	❑ Stock
❑ Iodine	❑ Milk Kefir	❑ Sunbathing	❑ Movement	❑ Ferments

Take a Moment:

I celebrate myself, and sing myself. —Walt Whitman

You have accomplished a lot! What do you celebrate in yourself?

_____

_____

_____

_____

Today's Focus: _____

Nutritional Intake:

Breakfast _____

Mid-morning_____

Lunch _____

Mid-afternoon _____

Dinner _____

Evening _____

New Foods/Reactions:_____

Stools (amount, number and type): _____

Quick Symptoms Checklist: **Rate Symptoms 0-10**

❑ Headache	❑ Digestive symptoms	Energy level:_____
❑ Joint pain	❑ Abdominal pain	Mood: _____
❑ Muscle pain	❑ Tinnitus	Mental Clarity:_____
❑ Other: _____	❑ Other: _____	Purpose/Hope: _____

My week overall: 0---10

I would describe my week (in one word) as: _____

Because? _____

General progress:

Advanced to a new stage? Y/N   Current stage?_____

New foods tolerated: _____   Foods removed: _____

Animal fats consumed: _____   Avg. daily amount: _____

# of days stock consumed: _____   Avg. daily amount: _____

Probiotics/fermented foods/cultured dairy:

Probiotic supplement: _____Current dose: _____

Die-off symptoms: Y/N   Describe: _____

_____

Beet Kvass_____   Sour Cream_____

Veggie Medley_____   Yogurt _____

Sauerkraut_____   Kefir_____

Detoxing Progress:

# of detox baths: _____ Ingredients: ACV/Epsom/Baking soda

# of days sunbathed: _____ # of minutes per session:_____ minutes

# of days juiced in am: _____in pm: _____

Ingredients:_____

Overall reactions to detoxing: _____

Symptoms descriptions:

Stools: Daily Y/N   #per day _____   Type(s):_____

Digestion: _____

Mood/energy: _____

Memory/clarity: _____

Sleep/Stress: _____

Typical-for-me symptoms: _____

_____

Date _____

❑ FCLO/HVBO	❑ Probiotic	❑ Detox Bath	❑ AM Juicing	❑ Fat
❑ Omega 3/6	❑ Beet Kvass	❑ Oil Pull	❑ PM Juicing	❑ Stock
❑ Iodine	❑ Milk Kefir	❑ Sunbathing	❑ Movement	❑ Ferments

Take a Moment:

Everything has beauty, but not everyone sees it. —Confucius

Take time to see the beauty around you. What did you see?

_____

_____

_____

_____

Today's Focus: _____

Nutritional Intake:

Breakfast _____

Mid-morning _____

Lunch _____

Mid-afternoon _____

Dinner _____

Evening _____

New Foods/Reactions: _____

Stools (amount, number and type): _____

_____

Quick Symptoms Checklist:		**Rate Symptoms 0-10**
❑ Headache	❑ Digestive symptoms	Energy level: _____
❑ Joint pain	❑ Abdominal pain	Mood: _____
❑ Muscle pain	❑ Tinnitus	Mental Clarity: _____
❑ Other: _____	❑ Other: _____	Purpose/Hope: _____

Date _____

❑ FCLO/HVBO	❑ Probiotic	❑ Detox Bath	❑ AM Juicing	❑ Fat
❑ Omega 3/6	❑ Beet Kvass	❑ Oil Pull	❑ PM Juicing	❑ Stock
❑ Iodine	❑ Milk Kefir	❑ Sunbathing	❑ Movement	❑ Ferments

Take a Moment:

Whenever you're making an important decision, first ask if it gets you closer to your goals or farther away. —Jillian Michaels

Take a minute today to remember and write down your goals.

_____

_____

_____

Today's Focus: _____

Nutritional Intake:

Breakfast _____

Mid-morning _____

Lunch _____

Mid-afternoon _____

Dinner _____

Evening _____

New Foods/Reactions: _____

Stools (amount, number and type): _____

Quick Symptoms Checklist: **Rate Symptoms 0-10**

❑ Headache	❑ Digestive symptoms	Energy level:_____
❑ Joint pain	❑ Abdominal pain	Mood: _____
❑ Muscle pain	❑ Tinnitus	Mental Clarity:_____
❑ Other: _____	❑ Other: _____	Purpose/Hope:____

Date _____

❏ FCLO/HVBO	❏ Probiotic	❏ Detox Bath	❏ AM Juicing	❏ Fat
❏ Omega 3/6	❏ Beet Kvass	❏ Oil Pull	❏ PM Juicing	❏ Stock
❏ Iodine	❏ Milk Kefir	❏ Sunbathing	❏ Movement	❏ Ferments

Take a Moment:

The greatest wealth is health. —Virgil

Health is a great goal to have! What is one area of health that you really want to work toward?

_____

_____

_____

Today's Focus: _____

Nutritional Intake:

Breakfast _____

Mid-morning _____

Lunch _____

Mid-afternoon _____

Dinner _____

Evening _____

New Foods/Reactions: _____

Stools (amount, number and type): _____

Quick Symptoms Checklist: **Rate Symptoms 0-10**

❏ Headache	❏ Digestive symptoms	Energy level:_____
❏ Joint pain	❏ Abdominal pain	Mood: _____
❏ Muscle pain	❏ Tinnitus	Mental Clarity:_____
❏ Other: _____	❏ Other: _____	Purpose/Hope: _____

Date _____

❏ FCLO/HVBO	❏ Probiotic	❏ Detox Bath	❏ AM Juicing	❏ Fat
❏ Omega 3/6	❏ Beet Kvass	❏ Oil Pull	❏ PM Juicing	❏ Stock
❏ Iodine	❏ Milk Kefir	❏ Sunbathing	❏ Movement	❏ Ferments

Take a Moment:

If you have only one smile in you, give it to the people you love.
Don't be surley at home, then go out in the street and start grinning
'Good morning' at total strangers. —Maya Angelou

Do the people at home get your love and kindness?

_____

_____

_____

Today's Focus: _____

Nutritional Intake:

Breakfast _____

Mid-morning_____

Lunch _____

Mid-afternoon _____

Dinner _____

Evening _____

New Foods/Reactions: _____

Stools (amount, number and type): _____

Quick Symptoms Checklist: Rate Symptoms 0-10

❏ Headache	❏ Digestive symptoms	Energy level:_____
❏ Joint pain	❏ Abdominal pain	Mood: _____
❏ Muscle pain	❏ Tinnitus	Mental Clarity:_____
❏ Other: _____	❏ Other: _____	Purpose/Hope: ____

Date _____

❑ FCLO/HVBO	❑ Probiotic	❑ Detox Bath	❑ AM Juicing	❑ Fat
❑ Omega 3/6	❑ Beet Kvass	❑ Oil Pull	❑ PM Juicing	❑ Stock
❑ Iodine	❑ Milk Kefir	❑ Sunbathing	❑ Movement	❑ Ferments

Take a Moment:

*Worry does not empty tomorrow of its sorrow,
it empties today of its strength.* —Corrie ten Boom

What are you worrying about today?

_____

_____

_____

Today's Focus: _____

Nutritional Intake:

Breakfast _____

Mid-morning_____

Lunch _____

Mid-afternoon _____

Dinner _____

Evening _____

New Foods/Reactions: _____

Stools (amount, number and type): _____

Quick Symptoms Checklist: **Rate Symptoms 0-10**

❑ Headache	❑ Digestive symptoms	Energy level:_____
❑ Joint pain	❑ Abdominal pain	Mood: _____
❑ Muscle pain	❑ Tinnitus	Mental Clarity: _____
❑ Other: _____	❑ Other: _____	Purpose/Hope: _____

Date _____

❑ FCLO/HVBO	❑ Probiotic	❑ Detox Bath	❑ AM Juicing	❑ Fat
❑ Omega 3/6	❑ Beet Kvass	❑ Oil Pull	❑ PM Juicing	❑ Stock
❑ Iodine	❑ Milk Kefir	❑ Sunbathing	❑ Movement	❑ Ferments

Take a Moment:

There is nothing sweeter than to be sympathized with. —George Santayana

When did someone sympathize with you?
How did that make you feel?

_____

_____

_____

Today's Focus: _____

Nutritional Intake:

Breakfast _____

Mid-morning _____

Lunch _____

Mid-afternoon _____

Dinner _____

Evening _____

New Foods/Reactions: _____

Stools (amount, number and type): _____

Quick Symptoms Checklist: **Rate Symptoms 0-10**

❑ Headache	❑ Digestive symptoms	Energy level:_____
❑ Joint pain	❑ Abdominal pain	Mood: _____
❑ Muscle pain	❑ Tinnitus	Mental Clarity:_____
❑ Other: _____	❑ Other: _____	Purpose/Hope: _____

Date _____

❑ FCLO/HVBO	❑ Probiotic	❑ Detox Bath	❑ AM Juicing	❑ Fat
❑ Omega 3/6	❑ Beet Kvass	❑ Oil Pull	❑ PM Juicing	❑ Stock
❑ Iodine	❑ Milk Kefir	❑ Sunbathing	❑ Movement	❑ Ferments

Take a Moment:

I am beginning to learn that it is the sweet, simple things of life which are the real ones after all. —Laura Ingalls Wilder

Write down the sweet things that you love in your life.

_____

_____

_____

Today's Focus: _____

Nutritional Intake:

Breakfast _____

Mid-morning _____

Lunch _____

Mid-afternoon _____

Dinner _____

Evening _____

New Foods/Reactions: _____

Stools (amount, number and type): _____

_____

Quick Symptoms Checklist:		Rate Symptoms 0-10
❑ Headache	❑ Digestive symptoms	Energy level:_____
❑ Joint pain	❑ Abdominal pain	Mood: _____
❑ Muscle pain	❑ Tinnitus	Mental Clarity:_____
❑ Other: _____	❑ Other: _____	Purpose/Hope: _____

My week overall: 0--10

I would describe my week (in one word) as: _____

Because? _____

General progress:

Advanced to a new stage? Y/N   Current stage?_____

New foods tolerated: _____   Foods removed: _____

Animal fats consumed: _____   Avg. daily amount: _____

# of days stock consumed: _____   Avg. daily amount: _____

Probiotics/fermented foods/cultured dairy:

Probiotic supplement: _____Current dose: _____

Die-off symptoms: Y/N   Describe: _____

_____

Beet Kvass _____   Sour Cream_____

Veggie Medley_____   Yogurt _____

Sauerkraut_____   Kefir_____

Detoxing Progress:

# of detox baths: _____ Ingredients: ACV/Epsom/Baking soda

# of days sunbathed: _____ # of minutes per session:_____ minutes

# of days juiced in am: _____in pm: _____

Ingredients:_____

Overall reactions to detoxing: _____

Symptoms descriptions:

Stools: Daily Y/N   #per day _____   Type(s):_____

Digestion: _____

Mood/energy: _____

Memory/clarity: _____

Sleep/Stress: _____

Typical-for-me symptoms: _____

_____

Date _____

❑ FCLO/HVBO	❑ Probiotic	❑ Detox Bath	❑ AM Juicing	❑ Fat
❑ Omega 3/6	❑ Beet Kvass	❑ Oil Pull	❑ PM Juicing	❑ Stock
❑ Iodine	❑ Milk Kefir	❑ Sunbathing	❑ Movement	❑ Ferments

Take a Moment:

Don't focus on the minutia of life. When you come to a wall in the road, life is telling you to make a turn. Go for it. —Howard Murad

This is a great perspective. Do you need it somewhere today?

_____

_____

_____

Today's Focus: _____

Nutritional Intake:

Breakfast _____

Mid-morning _____

Lunch _____

Mid-afternoon _____

Dinner _____

Evening _____

New Foods/Reactions: _____

Stools (amount, number and type): _____

Quick Symptoms Checklist: **Rate Symptoms 0-10**

❑ Headache	❑ Digestive symptoms	Energy level:_____
❑ Joint pain	❑ Abdominal pain	Mood: _____
❑ Muscle pain	❑ Tinnitus	Mental Clarity:_____
❑ Other: _____	❑ Other: _____	Purpose/Hope:_____

Date _____

- ❏ FCLO/HVBO
- ❏ Omega 3/6
- ❏ Iodine
- ❏ Probiotic
- ❏ Beet Kvass
- ❏ Milk Kefir
- ❏ Detox Bath
- ❏ Oil Pull
- ❏ Sunbathing
- ❏ AM Juicing
- ❏ PM Juicing
- ❏ Movement
- ❏ Fat
- ❏ Stock
- ❏ Ferments

Take a Moment:

Man starts over again everyday, in spite of all he knows, against all he knows. —Emil Cioran

Does this encourage or discourage you?

_____

_____

_____

Today's Focus: _____

Nutritional Intake:

Breakfast _____

Mid-morning _____

Lunch _____

Mid-afternoon _____

Dinner _____

Evening _____

New Foods/Reactions: _____

Stools (amount, number and type): _____

_____

Quick Symptoms Checklist: **Rate Symptoms 0-10**

❏ Headache	❏ Digestive symptoms	Energy level:_____
❏ Joint pain	❏ Abdominal pain	Mood: _____
❏ Muscle pain	❏ Tinnitus	Mental Clarity:_____
❏ Other: _____	❏ Other: _____	Purpose/Hope:_____

315

Date _____

❑ FCLO/HVBO	❑ Probiotic	❑ Detox Bath	❑ AM Juicing	❑ Fat
❑ Omega 3/6	❑ Beet Kvass	❑ Oil Pull	❑ PM Juicing	❑ Stock
❑ Iodine	❑ Milk Kefir	❑ Sunbathing	❑ Movement	❑ Ferments

Take a Moment:

Healing is not an overnight process, it is a daily cleansing of pain, it is a daily healing of your life. —Leon Brown

Write your reaction to this quote.

_____

_____

_____

Today's Focus: _____

Nutritional Intake:

Breakfast _____

Mid-morning_____

Lunch _____

Mid-afternoon _____

Dinner _____

Evening _____

New Foods/Reactions: _____

Stools (amount, number and type): _____

Quick Symptoms Checklist: **Rate Symptoms 0-10**

❑ Headache	❑ Digestive symptoms	Energy level:_____
❑ Joint pain	❑ Abdominal pain	Mood: _____
❑ Muscle pain	❑ Tinnitus	Mental Clarity:_____
❑ Other: _____	❑ Other: _____	Purpose/Hope:_____

Date _____

❏ FCLO/HVBO	❏ Probiotic	❏ Detox Bath	❏ AM Juicing	❏ Fat
❏ Omega 3/6	❏ Beet Kvass	❏ Oil Pull	❏ PM Juicing	❏ Stock
❏ Iodine	❏ Milk Kefir	❏ Sunbathing	❏ Movement	❏ Ferments

Take a Moment:

Food for the body is not enough. There must be food for the soul.
—Dorothy Day

What feeds your soul? How often do you partake of it?

_____

_____

_____

Today's Focus: _____

Nutritional Intake:

Breakfast _____

Mid-morning _____

Lunch _____

Mid-afternoon _____

Dinner _____

Evening _____

New Foods/Reactions: _____

Stools (amount, number and type): _____

Quick Symptoms Checklist: **Rate Symptoms 0-10**

❏ Headache	❏ Digestive symptoms	Energy level: _____
❏ Joint pain	❏ Abdominal pain	Mood: _____
❏ Muscle pain	❏ Tinnitus	Mental Clarity: _____
❏ Other: _____	❏ Other: _____	Purpose/Hope: _____

Date _____

❑ FCLO/HVBO	❑ Probiotic	❑ Detox Bath	❑ AM Juicing	❑ Fat
❑ Omega 3/6	❑ Beet Kvass	❑ Oil Pull	❑ PM Juicing	❑ Stock
❑ Iodine	❑ Milk Kefir	❑ Sunbathing	❑ Movement	❑ Ferments

Take a Moment:

We promise according to our hopes and perform according to our fears.
—Francios de La Rochefoucauld

Can you tell when you are believing in your hopes and when you are believing in your fears?

_____

_____

_____

Today's Focus: _____

Nutritional Intake:

Breakfast _____

Mid-morning _____

Lunch _____

Mid-afternoon _____

Dinner _____

Evening _____

New Foods/Reactions: _____

Stools (amount, number and type): _____

Quick Symptoms Checklist: **Rate Symptoms 0-10**

❑ Headache	❑ Digestive symptoms	Energy level:_____
❑ Joint pain	❑ Abdominal pain	Mood: _____
❑ Muscle pain	❑ Tinnitus	Mental Clarity:_____
❑ Other: _____	❑ Other: _____	Purpose/Hope: ____

Date _____

❏ FCLO/HVBO	❏ Probiotic	❏ Detox Bath	❏ AM Juicing	❏ Fat
❏ Omega 3/6	❏ Beet Kvass	❏ Oil Pull	❏ PM Juicing	❏ Stock
❏ Iodine	❏ Milk Kefir	❏ Sunbathing	❏ Movement	❏ Ferments

Take a Moment:

You are not your illness. You have an individual story to tell. You have a name, a history, a personality. Staying yourself is part of the battle.
—Julian Seifte

Who are you? Write down what makes you truely you.

_____

_____

_____

Today's Focus: _____

Nutritional Intake:

Breakfast _____

Mid-morning _____

Lunch _____

Mid-afternoon _____

Dinner _____

Evening _____

New Foods/Reactions: _____

Stools (amount, number and type): _____

Quick Symptoms Checklist: **Rate Symptoms 0-10**

❏ Headache	❏ Digestive symptoms	Energy level:_____
❏ Joint pain	❏ Abdominal pain	Mood: _____
❏ Muscle pain	❏ Tinnitus	Mental Clarity:_____
❏ Other: _____	❏ Other: _____	Purpose/Hope: ____

Date _____

❑ FCLO/HVBO	❑ Probiotic	❑ Detox Bath	❑ AM Juicing	❑ Fat
❑ Omega 3/6	❑ Beet Kvass	❑ Oil Pull	❑ PM Juicing	❑ Stock
❑ Iodine	❑ Milk Kefir	❑ Sunbathing	❑ Movement	❑ Ferments

Take a Moment:

Music is the unspoken language that can convey feelings more accurately than talking ever could. —Elizabeth Smart

Do you have feelings too deep to express by talking?
Can you find music to express them?

_____

_____

_____

Today's Focus: _____

Nutritional Intake:

Breakfast _____

Mid-morning _____

Lunch _____

Mid-afternoon _____

Dinner _____

Evening _____

New Foods/Reactions: _____

Stools (amount, number and type): _____

Quick Symptoms Checklist: **Rate Symptoms 0-10**

❑ Headache	❑ Digestive symptoms	Energy level:_____
❑ Joint pain	❑ Abdominal pain	Mood: _____
❑ Muscle pain	❑ Tinnitus	Mental Clarity: _____
❑ Other: _____	❑ Other: _____	Purpose/Hope: _____

My week overall: 0--10

I would describe my week (in one word) as: _____

Because? _____

General progress:

Advanced to a new stage? Y/N   Current stage?_____

New foods tolerated: _____   Foods removed: _____

Animal fats consumed: _____   Avg. daily amount: _____

# of days stock consumed: _____   Avg. daily amount: _____

Probiotics/fermented foods/cultured dairy:

Probiotic supplement: _____Current dose: _____

Die-off symptoms: Y/N   Describe: _____

_____

Beet Kvass _____   Sour Cream _____

Veggie Medley_____   Yogurt _____

Sauerkraut_____   Kefir_____

Detoxing Progress:

# of detox baths: _____ Ingredients: ACV/Epsom/Baking soda

# of days sunbathed: _____ # of minutes per session:_____ minutes

# of days juiced in am: _____in pm: _____

Ingredients:_____

Overall reactions to detoxing: _____

Symptoms descriptions:

Stools: Daily Y/N   #per day _____   Type(s):_____

Digestion: _____

Mood/energy: _____

Memory/clarity: _____

Sleep/Stress: _____

Typical-for-me symptoms: _____

_____

Date _____

❏ FCLO/HVBO	❏ Probiotic	❏ Detox Bath	❏ AM Juicing	❏ Fat
❏ Omega 3/6	❏ Beet Kvass	❏ Oil Pull	❏ PM Juicing	❏ Stock
❏ Iodine	❏ Milk Kefir	❏ Sunbathing	❏ Movement	❏ Ferments

Take a Moment:

The world is indeed full of peril, and in it there are many dark places; but still there is much that is fair, and though in all lands love is not mingled with grief, it grows perhaps the greater. —J.R.R. Tolkien

In your life, has your love become stronger because it has been mixed with grief?

_____

_____

Today's Focus: _____

Nutritional Intake:

Breakfast _____

Mid-morning_____

Lunch _____

Mid-afternoon _____

Dinner _____

Evening _____

New Foods/Reactions: _____

Stools (amount, number and type): _____

Quick Symptoms Checklist:		Rate Symptoms 0-10
❏ Headache	❏ Digestive symptoms	Energy level:_____
❏ Joint pain	❏ Abdominal pain	Mood: _____
❏ Muscle pain	❏ Tinnitus	Mental Clarity: _____
❏ Other: _____	❏ Other: _____	Purpose/Hope: _____

Date _____

❏ FCLO/HVBO	❏ Probiotic	❏ Detox Bath	❏ AM Juicing	❏ Fat
❏ Omega 3/6	❏ Beet Kvass	❏ Oil Pull	❏ PM Juicing	❏ Stock
❏ Iodine	❏ Milk Kefir	❏ Sunbathing	❏ Movement	❏ Ferments

Take a Moment:

I'm so glad I live in a world where there are Octobers. —L.M. Montgomery

We don't have to be thankful to special or detailed things. What are you just thankful for today?

_____

_____

_____

Today's Focus: _____

Nutritional Intake:

Breakfast _____

Mid-morning _____

Lunch _____

Mid-afternoon _____

Dinner _____

Evening _____

New Foods/Reactions: _____

Stools (amount, number and type): _____

Quick Symptoms Checklist: Rate Symptoms 0-10

❏ Headache	❏ Digestive symptoms	Energy level:_____
❏ Joint pain	❏ Abdominal pain	Mood: _____
❏ Muscle pain	❏ Tinnitus	Mental Clarity: _____
❏ Other: _____	❏ Other: _____	Purpose/Hope: _____

Date _____

❑ FCLO/HVBO	❑ Probiotic	❑ Detox Bath	❑ AM Juicing	❑ Fat
❑ Omega 3/6	❑ Beet Kvass	❑ Oil Pull	❑ PM Juicing	❑ Stock
❑ Iodine	❑ Milk Kefir	❑ Sunbathing	❑ Movement	❑ Ferments

Take a Moment:

Today is the first day of the rest of your life. —Abbie Hoffman

What do you want to do with the rest of your life?

_____

_____

_____

_____

Today's Focus: _____

Nutritional Intake:

Breakfast _____

Mid-morning _____

Lunch _____

Mid-afternoon _____

Dinner _____

Evening _____

New Foods/Reactions: _____

Stools (amount, number and type): _____

_____

Quick Symptoms Checklist: **Rate Symptoms 0-10**

❑ Headache	❑ Digestive symptoms	Energy level:_____
❑ Joint pain	❑ Abdominal pain	Mood: _____
❑ Muscle pain	❑ Tinnitus	Mental Clarity: _____
❑ Other: _____	❑ Other: _____	Purpose/Hope: _____

Date _____

Take a Moment:

> *Sometimes, carrying on, just carrying on,*
> *is the superhuman achievement.* —Albert Camus

Do you feel superhuman to just carry on?

_____

_____

_____

Today's Focus: _____

Nutritional Intake:

Breakfast _____

Mid-morning _____

Lunch _____

Mid-afternoon _____

Dinner _____

Evening _____

New Foods/Reactions: _____

Stools (amount, number and type): _____

Quick Symptoms Checklist: **Rate Symptoms 0-10**

❑ Headache   ❑ Digestive symptoms   Energy level:_____
❑ Joint pain   ❑ Abdominal pain   Mood: _____
❑ Muscle pain   ❑ Tinnitus   Mental Clarity:_____
❑ Other: _____   ❑ Other: _____   Purpose/Hope: _____

Date _____

❏ FCLO/HVBO	❏ Probiotic	❏ Detox Bath	❏ AM Juicing	❏ Fat
❏ Omega 3/6	❏ Beet Kvass	❏ Oil Pull	❏ PM Juicing	❏ Stock
❏ Iodine	❏ Milk Kefir	❏ Sunbathing	❏ Movement	❏ Ferments

Take a Moment:

Better to fight for something than live for nothing. —George S. Patton

Remind yourself what you are fighting for.

_____

_____

_____

_____

Today's Focus: _____

Nutritional Intake:

Breakfast _____

Mid-morning _____

Lunch _____

Mid-afternoon _____

Dinner _____

Evening _____

New Foods/Reactions: _____

Stools (amount, number and type): _____

Quick Symptoms Checklist: **Rate Symptoms 0-10**

❏ Headache	❏ Digestive symptoms	Energy level: _____
❏ Joint pain	❏ Abdominal pain	Mood: _____
❏ Muscle pain	❏ Tinnitus	Mental Clarity: _____
❏ Other: _____	❏ Other: _____	Purpose/Hope: _____

Date _____

❏ FCLO/HVBO	❏ Probiotic	❏ Detox Bath	❏ AM Juicing	❏ Fat
❏ Omega 3/6	❏ Beet Kvass	❏ Oil Pull	❏ PM Juicing	❏ Stock
❏ Iodine	❏ Milk Kefir	❏ Sunbathing	❏ Movement	❏ Ferments

Take a Moment:

Wit is the only wall between us and the dark. —Mark Van Doren

How has humor helped you in a dark situation?

_____

_____

_____

_____

Today's Focus: _____

Nutritional Intake:

Breakfast _____

Mid-morning_____

Lunch _____

Mid-afternoon _____

Dinner _____

Evening _____

New Foods/Reactions: _____

Stools (amount, number and type): _____

_____

Quick Symptoms Checklist: **Rate Symptoms 0-10**

❏ Headache	❏ Digestive symptoms	Energy level:_____
❏ Joint pain	❏ Abdominal pain	Mood: _____
❏ Muscle pain	❏ Tinnitus	Mental Clarity:_____
❏ Other: _____	❏ Other: _____	Purpose/Hope: _____

Date _____

❑ FCLO/HVBO	❑ Probiotic	❑ Detox Bath	❑ AM Juicing	❑ Fat
❑ Omega 3/6	❑ Beet Kvass	❑ Oil Pull	❑ PM Juicing	❑ Stock
❑ Iodine	❑ Milk Kefir	❑ Sunbathing	❑ Movement	❑ Ferments

Take a Moment:

Nothing we use or hear or touch can be expressed in words that equal what we are given by the senses. —Hannah Arendt

Spend time today enjoying the beauty around you, feeling things that you can't put into words.

_____

_____

_____

Today's Focus: _____

Nutritional Intake:

Breakfast _____

Mid-morning_____

Lunch _____

Mid-afternoon _____

Dinner _____

Evening _____

New Foods/Reactions: _____

Stools (amount, number and type): _____

Quick Symptoms Checklist: **Rate Symptoms 0-10**

❑ Headache	❑ Digestive symptoms	Energy level:_____
❑ Joint pain	❑ Abdominal pain	Mood: _____
❑ Muscle pain	❑ Tinnitus	Mental Clarity:_____
❑ Other: _____	❑ Other: _____	Purpose/Hope: _____

My week overall: 0---10

I would describe my week (in one word) as: _____

Because? _____

General progress:

Advanced to a new stage? Y/N   Current stage?_____

New foods tolerated: _____   Foods removed: _____

Animal fats consumed: _____   Avg. daily amount: _____

# of days stock consumed: _____   Avg. daily amount: _____

Probiotics/fermented foods/cultured dairy:

Probiotic supplement: _____Current dose: _____

Die-off symptoms: Y/N   Describe: _____

_____

Beet Kvass_____	Sour Cream_____
Veggie Medley_____	Yogurt _____
Sauerkraut_____	Kefir_____

Detoxing Progress:

# of detox baths: _____ Ingredients: ACV/Epsom/Baking soda

# of days sunbathed: _____ # of minutes per session:_____ minutes

# of days juiced in am: _____in pm: _____

Ingredients:_____

Overall reactions to detoxing: _____

Symptoms descriptions:

Stools: Daily Y/N   #per day _____   Type(s):_____

Digestion: _____

Mood/energy: _____

Memory/clarity: _____

Sleep/Stress: _____

Typical-for-me symptoms: _____

_____

Date _____

❑ FCLO/HVBO	❑ Prociotic	❑ Detox Bath	❑ AM Juicing	❑ Fat
❑ Omega 3/6	❑ Beet Kvass	❑ Oil Pull	❑ PM Juicing	❑ Stock
❑ Iodine	❑ Milk Kefir	❑ Sunbathing	❑ Movement	❑ Ferments

Take a Moment:

Wildness reminds us what it means to be human, what we are connected to rather than what we are separate from. —Terry Tempest Williams

Take time to be conneced today. Write your thoughts.

_____

_____

_____

Today's Focus: _____

Nutritional Intake:

Breakfast _____

Mid-morning _____

Lunch _____

Mid-afternoon _____

Dinner _____

Evening _____

New Foods/Reactions: _____

Stools (amount, number and type): _____

_____

Quick Symptoms Checklist: Rate Symptoms 0-10

❑ Headache	❑ Digestive symptoms	Energy level:_____
❑ Joint pain	❑ Abdominal pain	Moodiness:_____
❑ Muscle pain	❑ Tinnitus	Mental Clarity: _____
❑ Other: _____	❑ Other: _____	Purpose/Hope: _____

Date _____

❑ FCLO/HVBO	❑ Prociotic	❑ Detox Bath	❑ AM Juicing	❑ Fat
❑ Omega 3/6	❑ Beet Kvass	❑ Oil Pull	❑ PM Juicing	❑ Stock
❑ Iodine	❑ Milk Kefir	❑ Sunbathing	❑ Movement	❑ Ferments

Take a Moment:

Even if you fall on your face, you're still moving forward. —Victor Kiam

Write down how you are still moving forward, even today.

_____

_____

_____

_____

Today's Focus: _____

Nutritional Intake:

Breakfast _____

Mid-morning_____

Lunch _____

Mid-afternoon _____

Dinner _____

Evening _____

New Foods/Reactions: _____

Stools (amount, number and type): _____

Quick Symptoms Checklist: Rate Symptoms 0-10

❑ Headache	❑ Digestive symptoms	Energy level:_____
❑ Joint pain	❑ Abdominal pain	Moodiness:_____
❑ Muscle pain	❑ Tinnitus	Mental Clarity: _____
❑ Other: _____	❑ Other: _____	Purpose/Hope: _____

Date _____

❑ FCLO/HVBO	❑ Prociotic	❑ Detox Bath	❑ AM Juicing	❑ Fat
❑ Omega 3/6	❑ Beet Kvass	❑ Oil Pull	❑ PM Juicing	❑ Stock
❑ Iodine	❑ Milk Kefir	❑ Sunbathing	❑ Movement	❑ Ferments

Take a Moment:

The bad news is that yesterday sucked. The good news is that yesterday is gone. Today's a new day. Own it! Shape it! Live it! —Steve Maraboli

Did you have a bad day yesterday? It's over now. What are you going to do with today?

_____

_____

_____

Today's Focus: _____

Nutritional Intake:

Breakfast _____

Mid-morning _____

Lunch _____

Mid-afternoon _____

Dinner _____

Evening _____

New Foods/Reactions: _____

Stools (amount, number and type): _____

Quick Symptoms Checklist: Rate Symptoms 0-10

❑ Headache	❑ Digestive symptoms	Energy level:_____
❑ Joint pain	❑ Abdominal pain	Moodiness:_____
❑ Muscle pain	❑ Tinnitus	Mental Clarity:_____
❑ Other: _____	❑ Other: _____	Purpose/Hope:_____

Date _____

❑ FCLO/HVBO	❑ Prociotic	❑ Detox Bath	❑ AM Juicing	❑ Fat
❑ Omega 3/6	❑ Beet Kvass	❑ Oil Pull	❑ PM Juicing	❑ Stock
❑ Iodine	❑ Milk Kefir	❑ Sunbathing	❑ Movement	❑ Ferments

Take a Moment:

Do a little more each day than you think you possibly can.
—Lowell Thomas

I do not want you to exhaust yourself. But what is something you can do that is a little more than you think you can?

_____

_____

_____

Today's Focus: _____

Nutritional Intake:

Breakfast _____

Mid-morning_____

Lunch _____

Mid-afternoon _____

Dinner _____

Evening _____

New Foods/Reactions: _____

Stools (amount, number and type): _____

_____

Quick Symptoms Checklist: **Rate Symptoms 0-10**

❑ Headache	❑ Digestive symptoms	Energy level:_____
❑ Joint pain	❑ Abdominal pain	Moodiness:_____
❑ Muscle pain	❑ Tinnitus	Mental Clarity: _____
❑ Other: _____	❑ Other: _____	Purpose/Hope: _____

Date _____

❑ FCLO/HVBO	❑ Prociotic	❑ Detox Bath	❑ AM Juicing	❑ Fat
❑ Omega 3/6	❑ Beet Kvass	❑ Oil Pull	❑ PM Juicing	❑ Stock
❑ Iodine	❑ Milk Kefir	❑ Sunbathing	❑ Movement	❑ Ferments

Take a Moment:

I am doing the best I can given what I have today. —Jillian Michaels

Today comes with strengths and limitations. Are you okay to do your best, even if it's not what you wish you could do?

_____

_____

_____

Today's Focus: _____

Nutritional Intake:

Breakfast _____

Mid-morning _____

Lunch _____

Mid-afternoon _____

Dinner _____

Evening _____

New Foods/Reactions: _____

Stools (amount, number and type): _____

_____

Quick Symptoms Checklist: **Rate Symptoms 0-10**

❑ Headache	❑ Digestive symptoms	Energy level:_____
❑ Joint pain	❑ Abdominal pain	Moodiness:_____
❑ Muscle pain	❑ Tinnitus	Mental Clarity:_____
❑ Other: _____	❑ Other: _____	Purpose/Hope:_____

Date _____

❑ FCLO/HVBO	❑ Prociotic	❑ Detox Bath	❑ AM Juicing	❑ Fat
❑ Omega 3/6	❑ Beet Kvass	❑ Oil Pull	❑ PM Juicing	❑ Stock
❑ Iodine	❑ Milk Kefir	❑ Sunbathing	❑ Movement	❑ Ferments

Take a Moment:

> *Storms make trees take deeper roots.* —Dolly Parton

What roots have your storms deepened?

_____

_____

_____

_____

Today's Focus: _____

Nutritional Intake:

Breakfast _____

Mid-morning_____

Lunch _____

Mid-afternoon _____

Dinner _____

Evening _____

New Foods/Reactions: _____

Stools (amount, number and type): _____

Quick Symptoms Checklist: **Rate Symptoms 0-10**

❑ Headache	❑ Digestive symptoms	Energy level:_____
❑ Joint pain	❑ Abdominal pain	Moodiness:_____
❑ Muscle pain	❑ Tinnitus	Mental Clarity:_____
❑ Other: _____	❑ Other: _____	Purpose/Hope: ____

Date _____

❏ FCLO/HVBO	❏ Probiotic	❏ Detox Bath	❏ AM Juicing	❏ Fat
❏ Omega 3/6	❏ Beet Kvass	❏ Oil Pull	❏ PM Juicing	❏ Stock
❏ Iodine	❏ Milk Kefir	❏ Sunbathing	❏ Movement	❏ Ferments

Take a Moment:

Of all the diversions of life, there is none so proper to fill up its empty spaces as the reading of useful and entertaining authors.
—Joseph Addison

Do you read regularly? Spend some time in a book today!

_____

_____

_____

Today's Focus: _____

Nutritional Intake:

Breakfast _____

Mid-morning_____

Lunch _____

Mid-afternoon _____

Dinner _____

Evening _____

New Foods/Reactions:_____

Stools (amount, number and type): _____

Quick Symptoms Checklist: **Rate Symptoms 0-10**

❏ Headache	❏ Digestive symptoms	Energy level:_____
❏ Joint pain	❏ Abdominal pain	Mood: _____
❏ Muscle pain	❏ Tinnitus	Mental Clarity: _____
❏ Other: _____	❏ Other: _____	Purpose/Hope: ____

My week overall: 0---10

I would describe my week (in one word) as: _____

Because? _____

General progress:

Advanced to a new stage? Y/N   Current stage?_____

New foods tolerated: _____   Foods removed: _____

Animal fats consumed: _____   Avg. daily amount: _____

# of days stock consumed: _____   Avg. daily amount: _____

Probiotics/fermented foods/cultured dairy:

Probiotic supplement: _____Current dose: _____

Die-off symptoms: Y/N   Describe: _____

_____

Beet Kvass _____   Sour Cream _____

Veggie Medley_____   Yogurt _____

Sauerkraut_____   Kefir_____

Detoxing Progress:

# of detox baths: _____   Ingredients: ACV/Epsom/Baking soda

# of days sunbathed: _____   # of minutes per session:_____ minutes

# of days juiced in am: _____in pm: _____

Ingredients:_____

Overall reactions to detoxing: _____

Symptoms descriptions:

Stools: Daily Y/N   #per day _____   Type(s):_____

Digestion: _____

Mood/energy: _____

Memory/clarity: _____

Sleep/Stress: _____

Typical-for-me symptoms: _____

_____

Date _____

❏ FCLO/HVBO	❏ Probiotic	❏ Detox Bath	❏ AM Juicing	❏ Fat
❏ Omega 3/6	❏ Beet Kvass	❏ Oil Pull	❏ PM Juicing	❏ Stock
❏ Iodine	❏ Milk Kefir	❏ Sunbathing	❏ Movement	❏ Ferments

Take a Moment:

To achieve success, whatever the job we have, we must pay a price.
—Vince Lombardi

Think about the price you need to pay for a success. Are you ready to pay that price? If not, you need a new goal.

_____

_____

_____

Today's Focus: _____

Nutritional Intake:

Breakfast _____

Mid-morning_____

Lunch _____

Mid-afternoon _____

Dinner _____

Evening _____

New Foods/Reactions: _____

Stools (amount, number and type): _____

Quick Symptoms Checklist: **Rate Symptoms 0-10**

❏ Headache	❏ Digestive symptoms	Energy level:_____
❏ Joint pain	❏ Abdominal pain	Mood: _____
❏ Muscle pain	❏ Tinnitus	Mental Clarity: _____
❏ Other: _____	❏ Other: _____	Purpose/Hope: ____

Date _____

❏ FCLO/HVBO	❏ Probiotic	❏ Detox Bath	❏ AM Juicing	❏ Fat
❏ Omega 3/6	❏ Beet Kvass	❏ Oil Pull	❏ PM Juicing	❏ Stock
❏ Iodine	❏ Milk Kefir	❏ Sunbathing	❏ Movement	❏ Ferments

Take a Moment:

Each day is a blank page in the diary of your life. The secret of success is in turning that diary into the best story you possibly can.
—Douglas Pagels

Today is a new day, what story do you want to write in it?

_____

_____

_____

Today's Focus: _____

Nutritional Intake:

Breakfast _____

Mid-morning _____

Lunch _____

Mid-afternoon _____

Dinner _____

Evening _____

New Foods/Reactions: _____

Stools (amount, number and type): _____

Quick Symptoms Checklist: Rate Symptoms 0-10

❏ Headache	❏ Digestive symptoms	Energy level: _____
❏ Joint pain	❏ Abdominal pain	Mood: _____
❏ Muscle pain	❏ Tinnitus	Mental Clarity: _____
❏ Other: _____	❏ Other: _____	Purpose/Hope: _____

Date _____

❑ FCLO/HVBO	❑ Probiotic	❑ Detox Bath	❑ AM Juicing	❑ Fat
❑ Omega 3/6	❑ Beet Kvass	❑ Oil Pull	❑ PM Juicing	❑ Stock
❑ Iodine	❑ Milk Kefir	❑ Sunbathing	❑ Movement	❑ Ferments

Take a Moment:

Always be generous with your encouraging words, you may find they will inspire others to be the best they can be. —Catherine Pulsifer

How can you encourage someone today? Tell them!

_____

_____

_____

Today's Focus: _____

Nutritional Intake:

Breakfast _____

Mid-morning _____

Lunch _____

Mid-afternoon _____

Dinner _____

Evening _____

New Foods/Reactions: _____

Stools (amount, number and type): _____

_____

Quick Symptoms Checklist: **Rate Symptoms 0-10**

❑ Headache	❑ Digestive symptoms	Energy level:_____
❑ Joint pain	❑ Abdominal pain	Mood: _____
❑ Muscle pain	❑ Tinnitus	Mental Clarity: _____
❑ Other: _____	❑ Other: _____	Purpose/Hope: ____

Date _____

❑ FCLO/HVBO	❑ Probiotic	❑ Detox Bath	❑ AM Juicing	❑ Fat
❑ Omega 3/6	❑ Beet Kvass	❑ Oil Pull	❑ PM Juicing	❑ Stock
❑ Iodine	❑ Milk Kefir	❑ Sunbathing	❑ Movement	❑ Ferments

Take a Moment:

Everything that is done in this world is done with hope. —Martin Luther

Do you have hope today? What can you accomplish with that hope?

_____

_____

_____

Today's Focus: _____

Nutritional Intake:

Breakfast _____

Mid-morning _____

Lunch _____

Mid-afternoon _____

Dinner _____

Evening _____

New Foods/Reactions: _____

Stools (amount, number and type): _____

Quick Symptoms Checklist: **Rate Symptoms 0-10**

❑ Headache	❑ Digestive symptoms	Energy level:_____
❑ Joint pain	❑ Abdominal pain	Mood: _____
❑ Muscle pain	❑ Tinnitus	Mental Clarity: _____
❑ Other: _____	❑ Other: _____	Purpose/Hope: _____

Date _____

❏ FCLO/HVBO	❏ Probiotic	❏ Detox Bath	❏ AM Juicing	❏ Fat
❏ Omega 3/6	❏ Beet Kvass	❏ Oil Pull	❏ PM Juicing	❏ Stock
❏ Iodine	❏ Milk Kefir	❏ Sunbathing	❏ Movement	❏ Ferments

Take a Moment:

> *The greatest act of faith some days is to simply get up and face another day.* —Amy Gatliff

Sometimes every day is hard. Can you have faith to face another day today?

_____

_____

_____

Today's Focus: _____

Nutritional Intake:

Breakfast _____

Mid-morning _____

Lunch _____

Mid-afternoon _____

Dinner _____

Evening _____

New Foods/Reactions: _____

Stools (amount, number and type): _____

_____

Quick Symptoms Checklist:		**Rate Symptoms 0-10**
❏ Headache	❏ Digestive symptoms	Energy level: _____
❏ Joint pain	❏ Abdominal pain	Mood: _____
❏ Muscle pain	❏ Tinnitus	Mental Clarity: _____
❏ Other: _____	❏ Other: _____	Purpose/Hope: _____

Date _____

❑ FCLO/HVBO	❑ Probiotic	❑ Detox Bath	❑ AM Juicing	❑ Fat
❑ Omega 3/6	❑ Beet Kvass	❑ Oil Pull	❑ PM Juicing	❑ Stock
❑ Iodine	❑ Milk Kefir	❑ Sunbathing	❑ Movement	❑ Ferments

Take a Moment:

Do not follow where the path may lead. Go instead where there is no path and leave a trail. —Muriel Strode

You are not following the path—what trail are you leaving behind?

_____

_____

_____

Today's Focus: _____

Nutritional Intake:

Breakfast _____

Mid-morning_____

Lunch _____

Mid-afternoon _____

Dinner _____

Evening _____

New Foods/Reactions: _____

Stools (amount, number and type): _____

Quick Symptoms Checklist: Rate Symptoms 0-10

❑ Headache	❑ Digestive symptoms	Energy level:_____
❑ Joint pain	❑ Abdominal pain	Mood: _____
❑ Muscle pain	❑ Tinnitus	Mental Clarity:_____
❑ Other: _____	❑ Other: _____	Purpose/Hope: ____

Date _____

❏ FCLO/HVBO	❏ Probiotic	❏ Detox Bath	❏ AM Juicing	❏ Fat
❏ Omega 3/6	❏ Beet Kvass	❏ Oil Pull	❏ PM Juicing	❏ Stock
❏ Iodine	❏ Milk Kefir	❏ Sunbathing	❏ Movement	❏ Ferments

Take a Moment:

Live today. Not yesterday. Not tomorrow. Just today. Inhabit your moments. Don't rent them out to tomorrow. —Jerry Spinelli

How can you choose to live in your moments today? Is this hard for you?

_____

_____

_____

Today's Focus: _____

Nutritional Intake:

Breakfast _____

Mid-morning _____

Lunch _____

Mid-afternoon _____

Dinner _____

Evening _____

New Foods/Reactions: _____

Stools (amount, number and type): _____

_____

Quick Symptoms Checklist: **Rate Symptoms 0-10**

❏ Headache	❏ Digestive symptoms	Energy level:_____
❏ Joint pain	❏ Abdominal pain	Mood: _____
❏ Muscle pain	❏ Tinnitus	Mental Clarity: _____
❏ Other: _____	❏ Other: _____	Purpose/Hope: _____

My week overall: 0--10

I would describe my week (in one word) as: _____

Because? _____

General progress:

Advanced to a new stage? Y/N   Current stage?_____

New foods tolerated: _____   Foods removed: _____

Animal fats consumed: _____   Avg. daily amount: _____

# of days stock consumed: _____   Avg. daily amount: _____

Probiotics/fermented foods/cultured dairy:

Probiotic supplement: _____Current dose: _____

Die-off symptoms: Y/N   Describe: _____

_____

Beet Kvass _____   Sour Cream _____

Veggie Medley_____   Yogurt _____

Sauerkraut_____   Kefir_____

Detoxing Progress:

# of detox baths: _____ Ingredients: ACV/Epsom/Baking soda

# of days sunbathed: _____ # of minutes per session:_____ minutes

# of days juiced in am: _____in pm: _____

Ingredients:_____

Overall reactions to detoxing: _____

Symptoms descriptions:

Stools: Daily Y/N   #per day _____   Type(s):_____

Digestion: _____

Mood/energy: _____

Memory/clarity: _____

Sleep/Stress: _____

Typical-for-me symptoms: _____

_____

Date _____

❑ FCLO/HVBO	❑ Probiotic	❑ Detox Bath	❑ AM Juicing	❑ Fat
❑ Omega 3/6	❑ Beet Kvass	❑ Oil Pull	❑ PM Juicing	❑ Stock
❑ Iodine	❑ Milk Kefir	❑ Sunbathing	❑ Movement	❑ Ferments

Take a Moment:

You might not be the smartest, richest or best looking person but you're probably not the dumbest, ugliest or poorest either. —Rob Liano

You are you. What do you think about yourself?

_____

_____

_____

Today's Focus: _____

Nutritional Intake:

Breakfast _____

Mid-morning _____

Lunch _____

Mid-afternoon _____

Dinner _____

Evening _____

New Foods/Reactions: _____

Stools (amount, number and type): _____

Quick Symptoms Checklist: **Rate Symptoms 0-10**

❑ Headache	❑ Digestive symptoms	Energy level:_____
❑ Joint pain	❑ Abdominal pain	Mood: _____
❑ Muscle pain	❑ Tinnitus	Mental Clarity: _____
❑ Other: _____	❑ Other: _____	Purpose/Hope: _____

Date _____

☐ FCLO/HVBO   ☐ Probiotic   ☐ Detox Bath   ☐ AM Juicing   ☐ Fat
☐ Omega 3/6   ☐ Beet Kvass   ☐ Oil Pull   ☐ PM Juicing   ☐ Stock
☐ Iodine   ☐ Milk Kefir   ☐ Sunbathing   ☐ Movement   ☐ Ferments

Take a Moment:

The beginning is always today. —Mary Shelly

Does today feel like a new beginning to you? If not, can you change your perspective?

_____

_____

_____

Today's Focus: _____

Nutritional Intake:

Breakfast _____

Mid-morning _____

Lunch _____

Mid-afternoon _____

Dinner _____

Evening _____

New Foods/Reactions: _____

Stools (amount, number and type): _____

Quick Symptoms Checklist: **Rate Symptoms 0-10**

☐ Headache   ☐ Digestive symptoms   Energy level:_____
☐ Joint pain   ☐ Abdominal pain   Mood: _____
☐ Muscle pain   ☐ Tinnitus   Mental Clarity:_____
☐ Other: _____   ☐ Other: _____   Purpose/Hope: _____

Date _____

❏ FCLO/HVBO	❏ Probiotic	❏ Detox Bath	❏ AM Juicing	❏ Fat
❏ Omega 3/6	❏ Beet Kvass	❏ Oil Pull	❏ PM Juicing	❏ Stock
❏ Iodine	❏ Milk Kefir	❏ Sunbathing	❏ Movement	❏ Ferments

Take a Moment:

The greatest joys in life are found not only in what we do and feel, but also in our quiet hopes and labors for others. —Bryant McGill

What can you quietly do for someone today?

_____

_____

_____

Today's Focus: _____

Nutritional Intake:

Breakfast _____

Mid-morning _____

Lunch _____

Mid-afternoon _____

Dinner _____

Evening _____

New Foods/Reactions: _____

Stools (amount, number and type): _____

Quick Symptoms Checklist: **Rate Symptoms 0-10**

❏ Headache	❏ Digestive symptoms	Energy level:_____
❏ Joint pain	❏ Abdominal pain	Mood: _____
❏ Muscle pain	❏ Tinnitus	Mental Clarity: _____
❏ Other: _____	❏ Other: _____	Purpose/Hope: ____

Date _____

❑ FCLO/HVBO	❑ Probiotic	❑ Detox Bath	❑ AM Juicing	❑ Fat
❑ Omega 3/6	❑ Beet Kvass	❑ Oil Pull	❑ PM Juicing	❑ Stock
❑ Iodine	❑ Milk Kefir	❑ Sunbathing	❑ Movement	❑ Ferments

Take a Moment:

One can aquire everything in solitude except character. —Stendhal

Relationships can be hard. Is there someone who is currently building your character?

_____

_____

_____

Today's Focus: _____

Nutritional Intake:

Breakfast _____

Mid-morning_____

Lunch _____

Mid-afternoon _____

Dinner _____

Evening _____

New Foods/Reactions: _____

Stools (amount, number and type): _____

_____

Quick Symptoms Checklist: Rate Symptoms 0-10

❑ Headache	❑ Digestive symptoms	Energy level:_____
❑ Joint pain	❑ Abdominal pain	Mood: _____
❑ Muscle pain	❑ Tinnitus	Mental Clarity:_____
❑ Other: _____	❑ Other: _____	Purpose/Hope:_____

Date _____

❏ FCLO/HVBO	❏ Probiotic	❏ Detox Bath	❏ AM Juicing	❏ Fat
❏ Omega 3/6	❏ Beet Kvass	❏ Oil Pull	❏ PM Juicing	❏ Stock
❏ Iodine	❏ Milk Kefir	❏ Sunbathing	❏ Movement	❏ Ferments

Take a Moment:

Never give up, never surrender. —Galaxy Quest

Sometimes it just helps to repeat something short and silly–it just might becomes profoud. Write down any profound thoughts you have.

_____

_____

_____

Today's Focus: _____

Nutritional Intake:

Breakfast _____

Mid-morning _____

Lunch _____

Mid-afternoon _____

Dinner _____

Evening _____

New Foods/Reactions: _____

Stools (amount, number and type): _____

Quick Symptoms Checklist: **Rate Symptoms 0-10**

❏ Headache	❏ Digestive symptoms	Energy level:_____
❏ Joint pain	❏ Abdominal pain	Mood: _____
❏ Muscle pain	❏ Tinnitus	Mental Clarity: _____
❏ Other: _____	❏ Other: _____	Purpose/Hope: _____

Date _____

- ❑ FCLO/HVBO
- ❑ Omega 3/6
- ❑ Iodine
- ❑ Probiotic
- ❑ Beet Kvass
- ❑ Milk Kefir
- ❑ Detox Bath
- ❑ Oil Pull
- ❑ Sunbathing
- ❑ AM Juicing
- ❑ PM Juicing
- ❑ Movement
- ❑ Fat
- ❑ Stock
- ❑ Ferments

Take a Moment:

New beginnings are often disguised as painful endings. —Lao Tzu

Share a painful ending that was actually a new beginning.

_____
_____
_____
_____

Today's Focus: _____

Nutritional Intake:

Breakfast _____

Mid-morning _____

Lunch _____

Mid-afternoon _____

Dinner _____

Evening _____

New Foods/Reactions: _____

Stools (amount, number and type): _____

_____

Quick Symptoms Checklist: **Rate Symptoms 0-10**

- ❑ Headache
- ❑ Joint pain
- ❑ Muscle pain
- ❑ Other: _____

- ❑ Digestive symptoms
- ❑ Abdominal pain
- ❑ Tinnitus
- ❑ Other: _____

Energy level: _____
Mood: _____
Mental Clarity: _____
Purpose/Hope: _____

Date _____

❑ FCLO/HVBO	❑ Probiotic	❑ Detox Bath	❑ AM Juicing	❑ Fat
❑ Omega 3/6	❑ Beet Kvass	❑ Oil Pull	❑ PM Juicing	❑ Stock
❑ Iodine	❑ Milk Kefir	❑ Sunbathing	❑ Movement	❑ Ferments

Take a Moment:

Be soft. Do not let the world make you hate. Do not let the bitterness steal your sweetness. Take pride that even though the rest of the world may disagree, you still believe it to be a beautiful place. —Kurt Vonnegut, Jr.

Disease can harden us. How soft are you?

_____

_____

_____

Today's Focus: _____

Nutritional Intake:

Breakfast _____

Mid-morning_____

Lunch _____

Mid-afternoon _____

Dinner _____

Evening _____

New Foods/Reactions:_____

Stools (amount, number and type): _____

Quick Symptoms Checklist: **Rate Symptoms 0-10**

❑ Headache	❑ Digestive symptoms	Energy level:_____
❑ Joint pain	❑ Abdominal pain	Mood: _____
❑ Muscle pain	❑ Tinnitus	Mental Clarity: _____
❑ Other: _____	❑ Other: _____	Purpose/Hope: _____

My week overall: 0--10

I would describe my week (in one word) as: _____

Because? _____

General progress:

Advanced to a new stage? Y/N   Current stage?_____

New foods tolerated: _____   Foods removed: _____

Animal fats consumed: _____   Avg. daily amount: _____

# of days stock consumed: _____   Avg. daily amount: _____

Probiotics/fermented foods/cultured dairy:

Probiotic supplement: _____Current dose: _____

Die-off symptoms: Y/N   Describe: _____

_____

Beet Kvass _____   Sour Cream _____

Veggie Medley _____   Yogurt _____

Sauerkraut_____   Kefir_____

Detoxing Progress:

# of detox baths: _____ Ingredients: ACV/Epsom/Baking soda

# of days sunbathed: _____ # of minutes per session:_____ minutes

# of days juiced in am: _____in pm: _____

Ingredients:_____

Overall reactions to detoxing: _____

Symptoms descriptions:

Stools: Daily Y/N   #per day _____   Type(s):_____

Digestion: _____

Mood/energy: _____

Memory/clarity: _____

Sleep/Stress: _____

Typical-for-me symptoms: _____

_____

Date _____

❏ FCLO/HVBO	❏ Probiotic	❏ Detox Bath	❏ AM Juicing	❏ Fat
❏ Omega 3/6	❏ Beet Kvass	❏ Oil Pull	❏ PM Juicing	❏ Stock
❏ Iodine	❏ Milk Kefir	❏ Sunbathing	❏ Movement	❏ Ferments

Take a Moment:

I like this place and could willingly waste my time in it.
—William Shakespeare

Go to somewhere you like and "waste" some time there today.

_____

_____

_____

Today's Focus: _____

Nutritional Intake:

Breakfast _____

Mid-morning _____

Lunch _____

Mid-afternoon _____

Dinner _____

Evening _____

New Foods/Reactions: _____

Stools (amount, number and type): _____

Quick Symptoms Checklist: **Rate Symptoms 0-10**

❏ Headache	❏ Digestive symptoms	Energy level: _____
❏ Joint pain	❏ Abdominal pain	Mood: _____
❏ Muscle pain	❏ Tinnitus	Mental Clarity: _____
❏ Other: _____	❏ Other: _____	Purpose/Hope: _____

Date _____

❑ FCLO/HVBO	❑ Probiotic	❑ Detox Bath	❑ AM Juicing	❑ Fat
❑ Omega 3/6	❑ Beet Kvass	❑ Oil Pull	❑ PM Juicing	❑ Stock
❑ Iodine	❑ Milk Kefir	❑ Sunbathing	❑ Movement	❑ Ferments

Take a Moment:

There is no substitute for work. —Vince Lombardi

Are you trying to find an easy way, or magic pill to fix something? What work do you just need to do?

_____

_____

_____

Today's Focus: _____

Nutritional Intake:

Breakfast _____

Mid-morning _____

Lunch _____

Mid-afternoon _____

Dinner _____

Evening _____

New Foods/Reactions: _____

Stools (amount, number and type): _____

_____

Quick Symptoms Checklist: **Rate Symptoms 0-10**

❑ Headache	❑ Digestive symptoms	Energy level:_____
❑ Joint pain	❑ Abdominal pain	Mood: _____
❑ Muscle pain	❑ Tinnitus	Mental Clarity: _____
❑ Other: _____	❑ Other: _____	Purpose/Hope: _____

Date _____

❏ FCLO/HVBO	❏ Probiotic	❏ Detox Bath	❏ AM Juicing	❏ Fat
❏ Omega 3/6	❏ Beet Kvass	❏ Oil Pull	❏ PM Juicing	❏ Stock
❏ Iodine	❏ Milk Kefir	❏ Sunbathing	❏ Movement	❏ Ferments

Take a Moment:

Support and encouragement are found in the most unlikely places.
—Raquel Cepeda

Have you been surprised by encouragement? How did that feel?

_____

_____

_____

Today's Focus: _____

Nutritional Intake:

Breakfast _____

Mid-morning _____

Lunch _____

Mid-afternoon _____

Dinner _____

Evening _____

New Foods/Reactions: _____

Stools (amount, number and type): _____

_____

Quick Symptoms Checklist:		**Rate Symptoms 0-10**
❏ Headache	❏ Digestive symptoms	Energy level:_____
❏ Joint pain	❏ Abdominal pain	Mood: _____
❏ Muscle pain	❏ Tinnitus	Mental Clarity: _____
❏ Other: _____	❏ Other: _____	Purpose/Hope: _____

Date _____

- ❑ FCLO/HVBO
- ❑ Omega 3/6
- ❑ Iodine
- ❑ Probiotic
- ❑ Beet Kvass
- ❑ Milk Kefir
- ❑ Detox Bath
- ❑ Oil Pull
- ❑ Sunbathing
- ❑ AM Juicing
- ❑ PM Juicing
- ❑ Movement
- ❑ Fat
- ❑ Stock
- ❑ Ferments

Take a Moment:

> *Change, like healing, takes time.* —Veronica Roth

Do you feel like this is taking too much time? Write your thoughts.

_____

_____

_____

_____

Today's Focus: _____

Nutritional Intake:

Breakfast _____

Mid-morning _____

Lunch _____

Mid-afternoon _____

Dinner _____

Evening _____

New Foods/Reactions: _____

Stools (amount, number and type): _____

Quick Symptoms Checklist: **Rate Symptoms 0-10**

❑ Headache	❑ Digestive symptoms	Energy level:_____
❑ Joint pain	❑ Abdominal pain	Mood: _____
❑ Muscle pain	❑ Tinnitus	Mental Clarity:_____
❑ Other: _____	❑ Other: _____	Purpose/Hope: _____

Date _____

❏ FCLO/HVBO	❏ Probiotic	❏ Detox Bath	❏ AM Juicing	❏ Fat
❏ Omega 3/6	❏ Beet Kvass	❏ Oil Pull	❏ PM Juicing	❏ Stock
❏ Iodine	❏ Milk Kefir	❏ Sunbathing	❏ Movement	❏ Ferments

Take a Moment:

I'm thankful for laughter, except when milk comes out of my nose.
—Woody Allen

What "silly" thing are you thankful for?

_____

_____

_____

Today's Focus: _____

Nutritional Intake:

Breakfast _____

Mid-morning_____

Lunch _____

Mid-afternoon _____

Dinner _____

Evening _____

New Foods/Reactions:_____

Stools (amount, number and type): _____

Quick Symptoms Checklist: **Rate Symptoms 0-10**

❏ Headache	❏ Digestive symptoms	Energy level:_____
❏ Joint pain	❏ Abdominal pain	Mood: _____
❏ Muscle pain	❏ Tinnitus	Mental Clarity: _____
❏ Other: _____	❏ Other: _____	Purpose/Hope: _____

Date _____

❏ FCLO/HVBO	❏ Probiotic	❏ Detox Bath	❏ AM Juicing	❏ Fat
❏ Omega 3/6	❏ Beet Kvass	❏ Oil Pull	❏ PM Juicing	❏ Stock
❏ Iodine	❏ Milk Kefir	❏ Sunbathing	❏ Movement	❏ Ferments

Take a Moment:

It takes courage to grow up and become who you really are.
—E.E. Cummings

You were created to be well, but it takes courage to live this way. Write your thoughts about this.

_____

_____

_____

Today's Focus: _____

Nutritional Intake:

Breakfast _____

Mid-morning _____

Lunch _____

Mid-afternoon _____

Dinner _____

Evening _____

New Foods/Reactions: _____

Stools (amount, number and type): _____

Quick Symptoms Checklist: Rate Symptoms 0-10

❏ Headache	❏ Digestive symptoms	Energy level:_____
❏ Joint pain	❏ Abdominal pain	Mood: _____
❏ Muscle pain	❏ Tinnitus	Mental Clarity:_____
❏ Other: _____	❏ Other: _____	Purpose/Hope: _____

Date _____

❑ FCLO/HVBO	❑ Probiotic	❑ Detox Bath	❑ AM Juicing	❑ Fat
❑ Omega 3/6	❑ Beet Kvass	❑ Oil Pull	❑ PM Juicing	❑ Stock
❑ Iodine	❑ Milk Kefir	❑ Sunbathing	❑ Movement	❑ Ferments

Take a Moment:

The really idle man gets nowhere. The perpetually busy man does not get much further. —Sir Heneage Ogilivie

Balance is important. Do you need to make any adjustments?

_____

_____

_____

Today's Focus: _____

Nutritional Intake:

Breakfast _____

Mid-morning_____

Lunch _____

Mid-afternoon _____

Dinner _____

Evening _____

New Foods/Reactions: _____

Stools (amount, number and type): _____

Quick Symptoms Checklist: **Rate Symptoms 0-10**

❑ Headache	❑ Digestive symptoms	Energy level:_____
❑ Joint pain	❑ Abdominal pain	Mood: _____
❑ Muscle pain	❑ Tinnitus	Mental Clarity: _____
❑ Other: _____	❑ Other: _____	Purpose/Hope: _____

My week overall: 0--10

I would describe my week (in one word) as: _____

Because? _____

General progress:

Advanced to a new stage? Y/N   Current stage?_____

New foods tolerated: _____   Foods removed: _____

Animal fats consumed: _____   Avg. daily amount: _____

# of days stock consumed: _____   Avg. daily amount: _____

Probiotics/fermented foods/cultured dairy:

Probiotic supplement: _____Current dose: _____

Die-off symptoms: Y/N   Describe: _____

_____

Beet Kvass _____   Sour Cream _____

Veggie Medley_____   Yogurt _____

Sauerkraut_____   Kefir_____

Detoxing Progress:

# of detox baths: _____ Ingredients: ACV/Epsom/Baking soda

# of days sunbathed: _____ # of minutes per session:_____ minutes

# of days juiced in am: _____in pm: _____

Ingredients:_____

Overall reactions to detoxing: _____

Symptoms descriptions:

Stools: Daily Y/N   #per day _____   Type(s):_____

Digestion: _____

Mood/energy: _____

Memory/clarity: _____

Sleep/Stress: _____

Typical-for-me symptoms: _____

_____

Date _____

❑ FCLO/HVBO	❑ Probiotic	❑ Detox Bath	❑ AM Juicing	❑ Fat
❑ Omega 3/6	❑ Beet Kvass	❑ Oil Pull	❑ PM Juicing	❑ Stock
❑ Iodine	❑ Milk Kefir	❑ Sunbathing	❑ Movement	❑ Ferments

Take a Moment:

In all of living, have much fun and laughter. Life is to be enjoyed, not just endured. —Gordon B. Hinckley

This is not always easy, it is often a choice. Do you (at least sometimes) enjoy life?

_____

_____

_____

Today's Focus: _____

Nutritional Intake:

Breakfast _____

Mid-morning _____

Lunch _____

Mid-afternoon _____

Dinner _____

Evening _____

New Foods/Reactions: _____

Stools (amount, number and type): _____

Quick Symptoms Checklist: **Rate Symptoms 0-10**

❑ Headache	❑ Digestive symptoms	Energy level:_____
❑ Joint pain	❑ Abdominal pain	Mood: _____
❑ Muscle pain	❑ Tinnitus	Mental Clarity:_____
❑ Other: _____	❑ Other: _____	Purpose/Hope: _____

Date _____

- ❏ FCLO/HVBO
- ❏ Omega 3/6
- ❏ Iodine
- ❏ Probiotic
- ❏ Beet Kvass
- ❏ Milk Kefir
- ❏ Detox Bath
- ❏ Oil Pull
- ❏ Sunbathing
- ❏ AM Juicing
- ❏ PM Juicing
- ❏ Movement
- ❏ Fat
- ❏ Stock
- ❏ Ferments

Take a Moment:

Be willing to be a beginner every single morning. —Meister Eckhart

Do you think you should be an expert by now? What do you need to be okay to be a beginner in today?

_____

_____

_____

Today's Focus: _____

Nutritional Intake:

Breakfast _____

Mid-morning _____

Lunch _____

Mid-afternoon _____

Dinner _____

Evening _____

New Foods/Reactions: _____

Stools (amount, number and type): _____

Quick Symptoms Checklist: Rate Symptoms 0-10

❏ Headache	❏ Digestive symptoms	Energy level: _____
❏ Joint pain	❏ Abdominal pain	Mood: _____
❏ Muscle pain	❏ Tinnitus	Mental Clarity: _____
❏ Other: _____	❏ Other: _____	Purpose/Hope: _____

Date _____

❑ FCLO/HVBO	❑ Probiotic	❑ Detox Bath	❑ AM Juicing	❑ Fat
❑ Omega 3/6	❑ Beet Kvass	❑ Oil Pull	❑ PM Juicing	❑ Stock
❑ Iodine	❑ Milk Kefir	❑ Sunbathing	❑ Movement	❑ Ferments

Take a Moment:

Be happy in the moment, that's enough.
Each moment is all we need, not more. —Mother Teresa

Write about why you are happy in this moment.

_____

_____

_____

Today's Focus: _____

Nutritional Intake:

Breakfast _____

Mid-morning_____

Lunch _____

Mid-afternoon _____

Dinner _____

Evening _____

New Foods/Reactions:_____

Stools (amount, number and type): _____

Quick Symptoms Checklist: **Rate Symptoms 0-10**

❑ Headache	❑ Digestive symptoms	Energy level:_____
❑ Joint pain	❑ Abdominal pain	Mood: _____
❑ Muscle pain	❑ Tinnitus	Mental Clarity: _____
❑ Other: _____	❑ Other: _____	Purpose/Hope: _____

Date _____

❑ FCLO/HVBO	❑ Probiotic	❑ Detox Bath	❑ AM Juicing	❑ Fat
❑ Omega 3/6	❑ Beet Kvass	❑ Oil Pull	❑ PM Juicing	❑ Stock
❑ Iodine	❑ Milk Kefir	❑ Sunbathing	❑ Movement	❑ Ferments

Take a Moment:

Strength lies in differences, not in similarities —Stephen R. Covey

Do you dislike your differences. How are they actually strengths?

_____

_____

_____

_____

Today's Focus: _____

Nutritional Intake:

Breakfast _____

Mid-morning_____

Lunch _____

Mid-afternoon _____

Dinner _____

Evening _____

New Foods/Reactions: _____

Stools (amount, number and type): _____

Quick Symptoms Checklist: **Rate Symptoms 0-10**

❑ Headache	❑ Digestive symptoms	Energy level:_____
❑ Joint pain	❑ Abdominal pain	Mood: _____
❑ Muscle pain	❑ Tinnitus	Mental Clarity:_____
❑ Other: _____	❑ Other: _____	Purpose/Hope: _____

Date _____

❏ FCLO/HVBO	❏ Probiotic	❏ Detox Bath	❏ AM Juicing	❏ Fat
❏ Omega 3/6	❏ Beet Kvass	❏ Oil Pull	❏ PM Juicing	❏ Stock
❏ Iodine	❏ Milk Kefir	❏ Sunbathing	❏ Movement	❏ Ferments

Take a Moment:

At times our own light goes out and is rekindled by a spark from another person. Each of us has cause to think with deep gratitude of those who have lighted the flame within us. —Albert Schweitzer

Write about a time when someone relit your hope.

_____

_____

_____

Today's Focus: _____

Nutritional Intake:

Breakfast _____

Mid-morning _____

Lunch _____

Mid-afternoon _____

Dinner _____

Evening _____

New Foods/Reactions: _____

Stools (amount, number and type): _____

Quick Symptoms Checklist: **Rate Symptoms 0-10**

❏ Headache	❏ Digestive symptoms	Energy level:_____
❏ Joint pain	❏ Abdominal pain	Mood: _____
❏ Muscle pain	❏ Tinnitus	Mental Clarity: _____
❏ Other: _____	❏ Other: _____	Purpose/Hope: _____

Date _____

❑ FCLO/HVBO	❑ Probiotic	❑ Detox Bath	❑ AM Juicing	❑ Fat
❑ Omega 3/6	❑ Beet Kvass	❑ Oil Pull	❑ PM Juicing	❑ Stock
❑ Iodine	❑ Milk Kefir	❑ Sunbathing	❑ Movement	❑ Ferments

Take a Moment:

Life is a journey for us all. We all face trials. We all have ups and downs. All of us are human. But we are all masters of our fate. We are the ones who decide how we are going to react to life. —Elizabeth Smart

You, like all of us, have faced trials. How are you going to react to them?

_____

_____

_____

Today's Focus: _____

Nutritional Intake:

Breakfast _____

Mid-morning _____

Lunch _____

Mid-afternoon _____

Dinner _____

Evening _____

New Foods/Reactions: _____

Stools (amount, number and type): _____

Quick Symptoms Checklist: **Rate Symptoms 0-10**

❑ Headache	❑ Digestive symptoms	Energy level: _____
❑ Joint pain	❑ Abdominal pain	Mood: _____
❑ Muscle pain	❑ Tinnitus	Mental Clarity: _____
❑ Other: _____	❑ Other: _____	Purpose/Hope: _____

Date _____

❑ FCLO/HVBO	❑ Probiotic	❑ Detox Bath	❑ AM Juicing	❑ Fat
❑ Omega 3/6	❑ Beet Kvass	❑ Oil Pull	❑ PM Juicing	❑ Stock
❑ Iodine	❑ Milk Kefir	❑ Sunbathing	❑ Movement	❑ Ferments

Take a Moment:

They say time heals all wounds, but that presumes the source of the grief is finite. —Cassandra Clare

Illness can be a continuous source of grief. Take time to grieve today.

_____

_____

_____

Today's Focus: _____

Nutritional Intake:

Breakfast _____

Mid-morning _____

Lunch _____

Mid-afternoon _____

Dinner _____

Evening _____

New Foods/Reactions: _____

Stools (amount, number and type): _____

Quick Symptoms Checklist: **Rate Symptoms 0-10**

❑ Headache	❑ Digestive symptoms	Energy level:_____
❑ Joint pain	❑ Abdominal pain	Mood: _____
❑ Muscle pain	❑ Tinnitus	Mental Clarity:_____
❑ Other: _____	❑ Other: _____	Purpose/Hope: _____

My week overall: 0---10

I would describe my week (in one word) as: _____

Because? _____

General progress:

Advanced to a new stage? Y/N   Current stage?_____

New foods tolerated: _____   Foods removed: _____

Animal fats consumed: _____   Avg. daily amount: _____

# of days stock consumed: _____   Avg. daily amount: _____

Probiotics/fermented foods/cultured dairy:

Probiotic supplement: _____Current dose: _____

Die-off symptoms: Y/N   Describe: _____

_____

Beet Kvass _____   Sour Cream _____

Veggie Medley_____   Yogurt _____

Sauerkraut_____   Kefir_____

Detoxing Progress:

# of detox baths: _____   Ingredients: ACV/Epsom/Baking soda

# of days sunbathed: _____   # of minutes per session:_____ minutes

# of days juiced in am: _____in pm: _____

Ingredients:_____

Overall reactions to detoxing: _____

Symptoms descriptions:

Stools: Daily Y/N   #per day _____   Type(s):_____

Digestion: _____

Mood/energy: _____

Memory/clarity: _____

Sleep/Stress: _____

Typical-for-me symptoms: _____

_____

Date _____

❑ FCLO/HVBO	❑ Probiotic	❑ Detox Bath	❑ AM Juicing	❑ Fat
❑ Omega 3/6	❑ Beet Kvass	❑ Oil Pull	❑ PM Juicing	❑ Stock
❑ Iodine	❑ Milk Kefir	❑ Sunbathing	❑ Movement	❑ Ferments

Take a Moment:

Never give up and don't ask why because every situation does not need an answer. I'm a firm believer that I don't worry about anything I can't control. —Eric Davis

Do you have to have an answer for everything? Can you let it go?

_____

_____

_____

Today's Focus: _____

Nutritional Intake:

Breakfast _____

Mid-morning_____

Lunch _____

Mid-afternoon _____

Dinner _____

Evening _____

New Foods/Reactions: _____

Stools (amount, number and type): _____

_____

Quick Symptoms Checklist: **Rate Symptoms 0-10**

❑ Headache	❑ Digestive symptoms	Energy level:_____
❑ Joint pain	❑ Abdominal pain	Mood: _____
❑ Muscle pain	❑ Tinnitus	Mental Clarity:_____
❑ Other: _____	❑ Other: _____	Purpose/Hope: _____

Date _____

❑ FCLO/HVBO	❑ Probiotic	❑ Detox Bath	❑ AM Juicing	❑ Fat
❑ Omega 3/6	❑ Beet Kvass	❑ Oil Pull	❑ PM Juicing	❑ Stock
❑ Iodine	❑ Milk Kefir	❑ Sunbathing	❑ Movement	❑ Ferments

Take a Moment:

In life, we make the best decisions we can with the information we have on hand. —Agnes Kamara-Umunna

Don't get bogged down in old decisions.
With today's information, what will you decide to do?

_____

_____

_____

Today's Focus: _____

Nutritional Intake:

Breakfast _____

Mid-morning _____

Lunch _____

Mid-afternoon _____

Dinner _____

Evening _____

New Foods/Reactions: _____

Stools (amount, number and type): _____

Quick Symptoms Checklist: Rate Symptoms 0-10

❑ Headache	❑ Digestive symptoms	Energy level:_____
❑ Joint pain	❑ Abdominal pain	Mood: _____
❑ Muscle pain	❑ Tinnitus	Mental Clarity:_____
❑ Other: _____	❑ Other: _____	Purpose/Hope: ____

Date _____

❑ FCLO/HVBO	❑ Probiotic	❑ Detox Bath	❑ AM Juicing	❑ Fat
❑ Omega 3/6	❑ Beet Kvass	❑ Oil Pull	❑ PM Juicing	❑ Stock
❑ Iodine	❑ Milk Kefir	❑ Sunbathing	❑ Movement	❑ Ferments

Take a Moment:

Don't ruin a good day because of a bad yesterday. —Unknown

Do you have a hard time moving on from a bad day. What helps you to start fresh?

_____

_____

_____

Today's Focus: _____

Nutritional Intake:

Breakfast _____

Mid-morning _____

Lunch _____

Mid-afternoon _____

Dinner _____

Evening _____

New Foods/Reactions: _____

Stools (amount, number and type): _____

Quick Symptoms Checklist:		Rate Symptoms 0-10
❑ Headache	❑ Digestive symptoms	Energy level:_____
❑ Joint pain	❑ Abdominal pain	Mood: _____
❑ Muscle pain	❑ Tinnitus	Mental Clarity: _____
❑ Other: _____	❑ Other: _____	Purpose/Hope: _____

Date _____

❑ FCLO/HVBO	❑ Probiotic	❑ Detox Bath	❑ AM Juicing	❑ Fat
❑ Omega 3/6	❑ Beet Kvass	❑ Oil Pull	❑ PM Juicing	❑ Stock
❑ Iodine	❑ Milk Kefir	❑ Sunbathing	❑ Movement	❑ Ferments

Take a Moment:

Constant kindness can accomplish much.
As the sun makes ice melt, kindness causes misunderstanding,
mistrust, and hostility to evaporate. —Albert Schweitzer

Can you bring the sun of kindness into a situation today?

_____

_____

_____

Today's Focus: _____

Nutritional Intake:

Breakfast _____

Mid-morning_____

Lunch _____

Mid-afternoon _____

Dinner _____

Evening _____

New Foods/Reactions: _____

Stools (amount, number and type): _____

Quick Symptoms Checklist: **Rate Symptoms 0-10**

❑ Headache	❑ Digestive symptoms	Energy level:_____
❑ Joint pain	❑ Abdominal pain	Mood: _____
❑ Muscle pain	❑ Tinnitus	Mental Clarity:_____
❑ Other: _____	❑ Other: _____	Purpose/Hope: _____

Date _____

❏ FCLO/HVBO	❏ Probiotic	❏ Detox Bath	❏ AM Juicing	❏ Fat
❏ Omega 3/6	❏ Beet Kvass	❏ Oil Pull	❏ PM Juicing	❏ Stock
❏ Iodine	❏ Milk Kefir	❏ Sunbathing	❏ Movement	❏ Ferments

Take a Moment:

Adopt the pace of nature: her secret is patience. —Ralph Waldo Emerson

What do you need to be patient about today?

_____

_____

_____

Today's Focus: _____

Nutritional Intake:

Breakfast _____

Mid-morning_____

Lunch _____

Mid-afternoon _____

Dinner _____

Evening _____

New Foods/Reactions: _____

Stools (amount, number and type): _____

Quick Symptoms Checklist: **Rate Symptoms 0-10**

❏ Headache	❏ Digestive symptoms	Energy level:_____
❏ Joint pain	❏ Abdominal pain	Mood: _____
❏ Muscle pain	❏ Tinnitus	Mental Clarity: _____
❏ Other: _____	❏ Other: _____	Purpose/Hope: _____

Date _____

❏ FCLO/HVBO	❏ Probiotic	❏ Detox Bath	❏ AM Juicing	❏ Fat
❏ Omega 3/6	❏ Beet Kvass	❏ Oil Pull	❏ PM Juicing	❏ Stock
❏ Iodine	❏ Milk Kefir	❏ Sunbathing	❏ Movement	❏ Ferments

Take a Moment:

Be happy with what you have while working for what you want.
—Helen Keller

This is a hard thing to do—can you do it?

_____

_____

_____

Today's Focus: _____

Nutritional Intake:

Breakfast _____

Mid-morning _____

Lunch _____

Mid-afternoon _____

Dinner _____

Evening _____

New Foods/Reactions: _____

Stools (amount, number and type): _____

_____

Quick Symptoms Checklist: **Rate Symptoms 0-10**

❏ Headache	❏ Digestive symptoms	Energy level: _____
❏ Joint pain	❏ Abdominal pain	Mood: _____
❏ Muscle pain	❏ Tinnitus	Mental Clarity: _____
❏ Other: _____	❏ Other: _____	Purpose/Hope: _____

Date _____

❑ FCLO/HVBO	❑ Probiotic	❑ Detox Bath	❑ AM Juicing	❑ Fat
❑ Omega 3/6	❑ Beet Kvass	❑ Oil Pull	❑ PM Juicing	❑ Stock
❑ Iodine	❑ Milk Kefir	❑ Sunbathing	❑ Movement	❑ Ferments

Take a Moment:

> *Real strength is not just a condition of one's muscle,*
> *but a tenderness in one's spirit.* —McCallister Dodds

Is it easy for your spirit to be tender?

_____

_____

_____

Today's Focus: _____

Nutritional Intake:

Breakfast _____

Mid-morning _____

Lunch _____

Mid-afternoon _____

Dinner _____

Evening _____

New Foods/Reactions: _____

Stools (amount, number and type): _____

_____

Quick Symptoms Checklist: **Rate Symptoms 0-10**

❑ Headache	❑ Digestive symptoms	Energy level:_____
❑ Joint pain	❑ Abdominal pain	Mood: _____
❑ Muscle pain	❑ Tinnitus	Mental Clarity: _____
❑ Other: _____	❑ Other: _____	Purpose/Hope: _____

My week overall: 0--10

I would describe my week (in one word) as: _____

Because? _____

General progress:

Advanced to a new stage? Y/N   Current stage?_____

New foods tolerated: _____   Foods removed: _____

Animal fats consumed:_____   Avg. daily amount: _____

# of days stock consumed: _____   Avg. daily amount: _____

Probiotics/fermented foods/cultured dairy:

Probiotic supplement: _____Current dose: _____

Die-off symptoms: Y/N   Describe: _____

_____

Beet Kvass_____   Sour Cream_____

Veggie Medley_____   Yogurt _____

Sauerkraut_____   Kefir_____

Detoxing Progress:

# of detox baths: _____ Ingredients: ACV/Epsom/Baking soda

# of days sunbathed: _____ # of minutes per session:_____ minutes

# of days juiced in am: _____in pm: _____

Ingredients:_____

Overall reactions to detoxing: _____

Symptoms descriptions:

Stools: Daily Y/N   #per day _____   Type(s):_____

Digestion: _____

Mood/energy: _____

Memory/clarity: _____

Sleep/Stress: _____

Typical-for-me symptoms: _____

_____

Date _____

❑ FCLO/HVBO	❑ Probiotic	❑ Detox Bath	❑ AM Juicing	❑ Fat
❑ Omega 3/6	❑ Beet Kvass	❑ Oil Pull	❑ PM Juicing	❑ Stock
❑ Iodine	❑ Milk Kefir	❑ Sunbathing	❑ Movement	❑ Ferments

Take a Moment:

Nature is pleased with simplicity. And nature is no dummy.
—Isaac Newton

Observe the simplicity of nature today. Write your observations.

_____

_____

_____

Today's Focus: _____

Nutritional Intake:

Breakfast _____

Mid-morning _____

Lunch _____

Mid-afternoon _____

Dinner _____

Evening _____

New Foods/Reactions: _____

Stools (amount, number and type): _____

Quick Symptoms Checklist: **Rate Symptoms 0-10**

❑ Headache	❑ Digestive symptoms	Energy level:_____
❑ Joint pain	❑ Abdominal pain	Mood: _____
❑ Muscle pain	❑ Tinnitus	Mental Clarity:_____
❑ Other: _____	❑ Other: _____	Purpose/Hope: _____

Date _____

❏ FCLO/HVBO	❏ Probiotic	❏ Detox Bath	❏ AM Juicing	❏ Fat
❏ Omega 3/6	❏ Beet Kvass	❏ Oil Pull	❏ PM Juicing	❏ Stock
❏ Iodine	❏ Milk Kefir	❏ Sunbathing	❏ Movement	❏ Ferments

Take a Moment:

It's probably my job to tell you that life isn't fair, but I figure you already know that. So instead, I'll tell you that hope is precious, and you're right not to give up. —C.J. Redwine

Hope is precious—what precious hope are you clinging to today?

_____

_____

_____

Today's Focus: _____

Nutritional Intake:

Breakfast _____

Mid-morning_____

Lunch _____

Mid-afternoon _____

Dinner _____

Evening _____

New Foods/Reactions: _____

Stools (amount, number and type): _____

Quick Symptoms Checklist: **Rate Symptoms 0-10**

❏ Headache	❏ Digestive symptoms	Energy level:_____
❏ Joint pain	❏ Abdominal pain	Mood: _____
❏ Muscle pain	❏ Tinnitus	Mental Clarity: _____
❏ Other: _____	❏ Other: _____	Purpose/Hope: _____

Date _____

❏ FCLO/HVBO	❏ Probiotic	❏ Detox Bath	❏ AM Juicing	❏ Fat
❏ Omega 3/6	❏ Beet Kvass	❏ Oil Pull	❏ PM Juicing	❏ Stock
❏ Iodine	❏ Milk Kefir	❏ Sunbathing	❏ Movement	❏ Ferments

Take a Moment:

Thanksgiving, after all, is a word of action. —W.J. Cameron

Do you think you can choose to be thankful?

_____

_____

_____

_____

Today's Focus: _____

Nutritional Intake:

Breakfast _____

Mid-morning_____

Lunch _____

Mid-afternoon _____

Dinner _____

Evening _____

New Foods/Reactions: _____

Stools (amount, number and type): _____

Quick Symptoms Checklist: **Rate Symptoms 0-10**

❏ Headache	❏ Digestive symptoms	Energy level:_____
❏ Joint pain	❏ Abdominal pain	Mood: _____
❏ Muscle pain	❏ Tinnitus	Mental Clarity:_____
❏ Other: _____	❏ Other: _____	Purpose/Hope:_____

Date _____

❏ FCLO/HVBO	❏ Probiotic	❏ Detox Bath	❏ AM Juicing	❏ Fat
❏ Omega 3/6	❏ Beet Kvass	❏ Oil Pull	❏ PM Juicing	❏ Stock
❏ Iodine	❏ Milk Kefir	❏ Sunbathing	❏ Movement	❏ Ferments

Take a Moment:

If you made a list of all the things you could be thankful for, the list would undoubtedly be longer than your misfortunes. —Catherine Pulsifer

If you have time, make this list today.

_____

_____

_____

Today's Focus: _____

Nutritional Intake:

Breakfast _____

Mid-morning _____

Lunch _____

Mid-afternoon _____

Dinner _____

Evening _____

New Foods/Reactions: _____

Stools (amount, number and type): _____

Quick Symptoms Checklist: **Rate Symptoms 0-10**

❏ Headache	❏ Digestive symptoms	Energy level:_____
❏ Joint pain	❏ Abdominal pain	Mood: _____
❏ Muscle pain	❏ Tinnitus	Mental Clarity:_____
❏ Other: _____	❏ Other: _____	Purpose/Hope:_____

Date _____

❏ FCLO/HVBO	❏ Probiotic	❏ Detox Bath	❏ AM Juicing	❏ Fat
❏ Omega 3/6	❏ Beet Kvass	❏ Oil Pull	❏ PM Juicing	❏ Stock
❏ Iodine	❏ Milk Kefir	❏ Sunbathing	❏ Movement	❏ Ferments

Take a Moment:

Thanksgiving Day is a good day to recommit our energies to giving thanks and just giving. —Amy Grant

Will you do this today?

_____

_____

_____

Today's Focus: _____

Nutritional Intake:

Breakfast _____

Mid-morning_____

Lunch _____

Mid-afternoon _____

Dinner _____

Evening _____

New Foods/Reactions: _____

Stools (amount, number and type): _____

Quick Symptoms Checklist: **Rate Symptoms 0-10**

❏ Headache	❏ Digestive symptoms	Energy level:_____
❏ Joint pain	❏ Abdominal pain	Mood: _____
❏ Muscle pain	❏ Tinnitus	Mental Clarity: _____
❏ Other: _____	❏ Other: _____	Purpose/Hope: _____

Date _____

❏ FCLO/HVBO	❏ Probiotic	❏ Detox Bath	❏ AM Juicing	❏ Fat
❏ Omega 3/6	❏ Beet Kvass	❏ Oil Pull	❏ PM Juicing	❏ Stock
❏ Iodine	❏ Milk Kefir	❏ Sunbathing	❏ Movement	❏ Ferments

Take a Moment:

Our chief want is someone who will inspire us to be what we know we could be. —Ralph Waldo Emerson

Have you been inspired like this? Can you inspire someone else?

_____

_____

_____

Today's Focus: _____

Nutritional Intake:

Breakfast _____

Mid-morning _____

Lunch _____

Mid-afternoon _____

Dinner _____

Evening _____

New Foods/Reactions: _____

Stools (amount, number and type): _____

Quick Symptoms Checklist: **Rate Symptoms 0-10**

❏ Headache	❏ Digestive symptoms	Energy level:_____
❏ Joint pain	❏ Abdominal pain	Mood: _____
❏ Muscle pain	❏ Tinnitus	Mental Clarity:_____
❏ Other: _____	❏ Other: _____	Purpose/Hope: _____

Date _____

❑ FCLO/HVBO	❑ Probiotic	❑ Detox Bath	❑ AM Juicing	❑ Fat
❑ Omega 3/6	❑ Beet Kvass	❑ Oil Pull	❑ PM Juicing	❑ Stock
❑ Iodine	❑ Milk Kefir	❑ Sunbathing	❑ Movement	❑ Ferments

Take a Moment:

Every sunset is an opportunity to reset. —Richie Norton

Do you feel like a failure in any area? Tomorrow is a new day–give yourself permission to press the reset button.

_____

_____

_____

Today's Focus: _____

Nutritional Intake:

Breakfast _____

Mid-morning_____

Lunch _____

Mid-afternoon _____

Dinner _____

Evening _____

New Foods/Reactions: _____

Stools (amount, number and type): _____

Quick Symptoms Checklist: **Rate Symptoms 0-10**

❑ Headache	❑ Digestive symptoms	Energy level:_____
❑ Joint pain	❑ Abdominal pain	Mood: _____
❑ Muscle pain	❑ Tinnitus	Mental Clarity:_____
❑ Other: _____	❑ Other: _____	Purpose/Hope: ____

My week overall: 0--10

I would describe my week (in one word) as: _____

Because? _____

General progress:

Advanced to a new stage? Y/N   Current stage?_____

New foods tolerated: _____   Foods removed: _____

Animal fats consumed:_____   Avg. daily amount: _____

# of days stock consumed: _____   Avg. daily amount: _____

Probiotics/fermented foods/cultured dairy:

Probiotic supplement: _____Current dose: _____

Die-off symptoms: Y/N   Describe: _____

_____

Beet Kvass _____   Sour Cream _____

Veggie Medley_____   Yogurt _____

Sauerkraut_____   Kefir_____

Detoxing Progress:

# of detox baths: _____   Ingredients: ACV/Epsom/Baking soda

# of days sunbathed: _____   # of minutes per session:_____ minutes

# of days juiced in am: _____in pm: _____

Ingredients:_____

Overall reactions to detoxing: _____

Symptoms descriptions:

Stools: Daily Y/N   #per day _____   Type(s):_____

Digestion: _____

Mood/energy: _____

Memory/clarity: _____

Sleep/Stress: _____

Typical-for-me symptoms: _____

_____

Date _____

❑ FCLO/HVBO	❑ Probiotic	❑ Detox Bath	❑ AM Juicing	❑ Fat
❑ Omega 3/6	❑ Beet Kvass	❑ Oil Pull	❑ PM Juicing	❑ Stock
❑ Iodine	❑ Milk Kefir	❑ Sunbathing	❑ Movement	❑ Ferments

Take a Moment:

Silence is a true friend who never betrays. —Confucius

Take time to be silent today.

_____

_____

_____

_____

Today's Focus: _____

Nutritional Intake:

Breakfast _____

Mid-morning _____

Lunch _____

Mid-afternoon _____

Dinner _____

Evening _____

New Foods/Reactions: _____

Stools (amount, number and type): _____

Quick Symptoms Checklist: **Rate Symptoms 0-10**

❑ Headache	❑ Digestive symptoms	Energy level: _____
❑ Joint pain	❑ Abdominal pain	Mood: _____
❑ Muscle pain	❑ Tinnitus	Mental Clarity: _____
❑ Other: _____	❑ Other: _____	Purpose/Hope: _____

Date _____

❏ FCLO/HVBO	❏ Probiotic	❏ Detox Bath	❏ AM Juicing	❏ Fat
❏ Omega 3/6	❏ Beet Kvass	❏ Oil Pull	❏ PM Juicing	❏ Stock
❏ Iodine	❏ Milk Kefir	❏ Sunbathing	❏ Movement	❏ Ferments

Take a Moment:

A pessimist is someone who has forgotten the joy of beginning.
—Marty Rubin

How are you approaching today?
Are you excited for a new beginning?

_____

_____

_____

Today's Focus: _____

Nutritional Intake:

Breakfast _____

Mid-morning _____

Lunch _____

Mid-afternoon _____

Dinner _____

Evening _____

New Foods/Reactions: _____

Stools (amount, number and type): _____

Quick Symptoms Checklist: Rate Symptoms 0-10

❏ Headache	❏ Digestive symptoms	Energy level: _____
❏ Joint pain	❏ Abdominal pain	Mood: _____
❏ Muscle pain	❏ Tinnitus	Mental Clarity: _____
❏ Other: _____	❏ Other: _____	Purpose/Hope: _____

Date _____

❑ FCLO/HVBO	❑ Probiotic	❑ Detox Bath	❑ AM Juicing	❑ Fat
❑ Omega 3/6	❑ Beet Kvass	❑ Oil Pull	❑ PM Juicing	❑ Stock
❑ Iodine	❑ Milk Kefir	❑ Sunbathing	❑ Movement	❑ Ferments

Take a Moment:

Encouragement is like water to the soul, it makes everything grow.
—Chris Burkmenn

Can you water someone's soul today?

_____

_____

_____

Today's Focus: _____

Nutritional Intake:

Breakfast _____

Mid-morning _____

Lunch _____

Mid-afternoon _____

Dinner _____

Evening _____

New Foods/Reactions: _____

Stools (amount, number and type): _____

Quick Symptoms Checklist: **Rate Symptoms 0-10**

❑ Headache	❑ Digestive symptoms	Energy level:_____
❑ Joint pain	❑ Abdominal pain	Mood: _____
❑ Muscle pain	❑ Tinnitus	Mental Clarity:_____
❑ Other: _____	❑ Other: _____	Purpose/Hope: _____

Date _____

- ❑ FCLO/HVBO
- ❑ Omega 3/6
- ❑ Iodine
- ❑ Probiotic
- ❑ Beet Kvass
- ❑ Milk Kefir
- ❑ Detox Bath
- ❑ Oil Pull
- ❑ Sunbathing
- ❑ AM Juicing
- ❑ PM Juicing
- ❑ Movement
- ❑ Fat
- ❑ Stock
- ❑ Ferments

Take a Moment:

Your victory is right around the corner. Never give up. —Nicki Minaj

What will keep you going today?

_____

_____

_____

_____

Today's Focus: _____

Nutritional Intake:

Breakfast _____

Mid-morning _____

Lunch _____

Mid-afternoon _____

Dinner _____

Evening _____

New Foods/Reactions: _____

Stools (amount, number and type): _____

Quick Symptoms Checklist: **Rate Symptoms 0-10**

- ❑ Headache
- ❑ Joint pain
- ❑ Muscle pain
- ❑ Other: _____
- ❑ Digestive symptoms
- ❑ Abdominal pain
- ❑ Tinnitus
- ❑ Other: _____

Energy level: _____
Mood: _____
Mental Clarity: _____
Purpose/Hope: _____

Date _____

❑ FCLO/HVBO	❑ Probiotic	❑ Detox Bath	❑ AM Juicing	❑ Fat
❑ Omega 3/6	❑ Beet Kvass	❑ Oil Pull	❑ PM Juicing	❑ Stock
❑ Iodine	❑ Milk Kefir	❑ Sunbathing	❑ Movement	❑ Ferments

Take a Moment:

At the end of the day, your health is your responsibility.
—Jillian Michaels

Are you taking responsibility for your health, or passing it off onto someone else?

_____

_____

_____

Today's Focus: _____

Nutritional Intake:

Breakfast _____

Mid-morning_____

Lunch _____

Mid-afternoon _____

Dinner _____

Evening _____

New Foods/Reactions: _____

Stools (amount, number and type): _____

Quick Symptoms Checklist: **Rate Symptoms 0-10**

❑ Headache	❑ Digestive symptoms	Energy level:_____
❑ Joint pain	❑ Abdominal pain	Mood: _____
❑ Muscle pain	❑ Tinnitus	Mental Clarity: _____
❑ Other: _____	❑ Other: _____	Purpose/Hope: _____

Date _____

❑ FCLO/HVBO	❑ Probiotic	❑ Detox Bath	❑ AM Juicing	❑ Fat
❑ Omega 3/6	❑ Beet Kvass	❑ Oil Pull	❑ PM Juicing	❑ Stock
❑ Iodine	❑ Milk Kefir	❑ Sunbathing	❑ Movement	❑ Ferments

Take a Moment:

The good Lord gave you a body that can stand most anything. It's your mind you have to convince. —Vince Lombardi

What is your body persevering in that your mind wants to give up on?

_____

_____

_____

Today's Focus: _____

Nutritional Intake:

Breakfast _____

Mid-morning _____

Lunch _____

Mid-afternoon _____

Dinner _____

Evening _____

New Foods/Reactions: _____

Stools (amount, number and type): _____

Quick Symptoms Checklist: **Rate Symptoms 0-10**

❑ Headache	❑ Digestive symptoms	Energy level:_____
❑ Joint pain	❑ Abdominal pain	Mood: _____
❑ Muscle pain	❑ Tinnitus	Mental Clarity:_____
❑ Other: _____	❑ Other: _____	Purpose/Hope: _____

Date _____

❑ FCLO/HVBO	❑ Probiotic	❑ Detox Bath	❑ AM Juicing	❑ Fat
❑ Omega 3/6	❑ Beet Kvass	❑ Oil Pull	❑ PM Juicing	❑ Stock
❑ Iodine	❑ Milk Kefir	❑ Sunbathing	❑ Movement	❑ Ferments

Take a Moment:

Many people spend more time planning the next holiday than examining the self. —Joseph Rain

It's important to know yourself. Take some time to do this today.

_____

_____

_____

Today's Focus: _____

Nutritional Intake:

Breakfast _____

Mid-morning _____

Lunch _____

Mid-afternoon _____

Dinner _____

Evening _____

New Foods/Reactions: _____

Stools (amount, number and type): _____

Quick Symptoms Checklist: **Rate Symptoms 0-10**

❑ Headache	❑ Digestive symptoms	Energy level:_____
❑ Joint pain	❑ Abdominal pain	Mood: _____
❑ Muscle pain	❑ Tinnitus	Mental Clarity: _____
❑ Other: _____	❑ Other: _____	Purpose/Hope: _____

My week overall: 0--10

I would describe my week (in one word) as: _____

Because? _____

General progress:

Advanced to a new stage? Y/N   Current stage?_____

New foods tolerated: _____   Foods removed: _____

Animal fats consumed:_____   Avg. daily amount: _____

# of days stock consumed: _____   Avg. daily amount: _____

Probiotics/fermented foods/cultured dairy:

Probiotic supplement: _____Current dose: _____

Die-off symptoms: Y/N   Describe: _____

_____

Beet Kvass _____   Sour Cream _____

Veggie Medley_____   Yogurt _____

Sauerkraut_____   Kefir_____

Detoxing Progress:

# of detox baths: _____ Ingredients: ACV/Epsom/Baking soda

# of days sunbathed: _____ # of minutes per session:_____ minutes

# of days juiced in am: _____in pm: _____

Ingredients:_____

Overall reactions to detoxing: _____

Symptoms descriptions:

Stools: Daily Y/N   #per day _____   Type(s):_____

Digestion: _____

Mood/energy: _____

Memory/clarity: _____

Sleep/Stress: _____

Typical-for-me symptoms: _____

_____

Date _____

❑ FCLO/HVBO	❑ Probiotic	❑ Detox Bath	❑ AM Juicing	❑ Fat
❑ Omega 3/6	❑ Beet Kvass	❑ Oil Pull	❑ PM Juicing	❑ Stock
❑ Iodine	❑ Milk Kefir	❑ Sunbathing	❑ Movement	❑ Ferments

Take a Moment:

A true healer is the one who heals himself first so others can benefit from his own healing. —Hong Curley

Many of us are healers at heart, and taking time to heal ourselves can be hard, especially if it takes longer than we think. Can you continue to give yourself time to heal?

_____

_____

Today's Focus: _____

Nutritional Intake:

Breakfast _____

Mid-morning_____

Lunch _____

Mid-afternoon _____

Dinner _____

Evening _____

New Foods/Reactions: _____

Stools (amount, number and type): _____

Quick Symptoms Checklist: **Rate Symptoms 0-10**

❑ Headache	❑ Digestive symptoms	Energy level:_____
❑ Joint pain	❑ Abdominal pain	Mood: _____
❑ Muscle pain	❑ Tinnitus	Mental Clarity: _____
❑ Other: _____	❑ Other: _____	Purpose/Hope: _____

Date _____

❏ FCLO/HVBO	❏ Probiotic	❏ Detox Bath	❏ AM Juicing	❏ Fat
❏ Omega 3/6	❏ Beet Kvass	❏ Oil Pull	❏ PM Juicing	❏ Stock
❏ Iodine	❏ Milk Kefir	❏ Sunbathing	❏ Movement	❏ Ferments

Take a Moment:

As soon as healing takes place, go out and heal somebody else.
—Maya Angelou

An outward focus can help healing as well. Have you experienced healing in any area that you can share with someone else?

_____

_____

_____

Today's Focus: _____

Nutritional Intake:

Breakfast _____

Mid-morning _____

Lunch _____

Mid-afternoon _____

Dinner _____

Evening _____

New Foods/Reactions: _____

Stools (amount, number and type): _____

Quick Symptoms Checklist: **Rate Symptoms 0-10**

❏ Headache	❏ Digestive symptoms	Energy level: _____
❏ Joint pain	❏ Abdominal pain	Mood: _____
❏ Muscle pain	❏ Tinnitus	Mental Clarity: _____
❏ Other: _____	❏ Other: _____	Purpose/Hope: _____

Date _____

❑ FCLO/HVBO	❑ Probiotic	❑ Detox Bath	❑ AM Juicing	❑ Fat
❑ Omega 3/6	❑ Beet Kvass	❑ Oil Pull	❑ PM Juicing	❑ Stock
❑ Iodine	❑ Milk Kefir	❑ Sunbathing	❑ Movement	❑ Ferments

Take a Moment:

Night never has the last word. The dawn is always invincible.
—Hugh B. Brown

What do you feel like will never end?

_____

_____

_____

Today's Focus: _____

Nutritional Intake:

Breakfast _____

Mid-morning _____

Lunch _____

Mid-afternoon _____

Dinner _____

Evening _____

New Foods/Reactions: _____

Stools (amount, number and type): _____

Quick Symptoms Checklist: **Rate Symptoms 0-10**

❑ Headache	❑ Digestive symptoms	Energy level:_____
❑ Joint pain	❑ Abdominal pain	Mood: _____
❑ Muscle pain	❑ Tinnitus	Mental Clarity:_____
❑ Other: _____	❑ Other: _____	Purpose/Hope: _____

Date _____

❑ FCLO/HVBO	❑ Probiotic	❑ Detox Bath	❑ AM Juicing	❑ Fat
❑ Omega 3/6	❑ Beet Kvass	❑ Oil Pull	❑ PM Juicing	❑ Stock
❑ Iodine	❑ Milk Kefir	❑ Sunbathing	❑ Movement	❑ Ferments

Take a Moment:

Once you learn to quit, it becomes a habit. —Vince Lombardi

Do you have the habit of quitting in anything?
Like all other habits, it can be broken.

_____

_____

_____

Today's Focus: _____

Nutritional Intake:

Breakfast _____

Mid-morning _____

Lunch _____

Mid-afternoon _____

Dinner _____

Evening _____

New Foods/Reactions: _____

Stools (amount, number and type): _____

Quick Symptoms Checklist: **Rate Symptoms 0-10**

❑ Headache	❑ Digestive symptoms	Energy level:_____
❑ Joint pain	❑ Abdominal pain	Mood: _____
❑ Muscle pain	❑ Tinnitus	Mental Clarity:_____
❑ Other: _____	❑ Other: _____	Purpose/Hope: _____

Date _____

❏ FCLO/HVBO	❏ Probiotic	❏ Detox Bath	❏ AM Juicing	❏ Fat
❏ Omega 3/6	❏ Beet Kvass	❏ Oil Pull	❏ PM Juicing	❏ Stock
❏ Iodine	❏ Milk Kefir	❏ Sunbathing	❏ Movement	❏ Ferments

Take a Moment:

Feelings follow actions. —Roxanne Henke

You don't have to wait for the feeling. Start the action of smiling or laughing–feelings will follow. What feeling do you want today?

_____

_____

_____

Today's Focus: _____

Nutritional Intake:

Breakfast _____

Mid-morning_____

Lunch _____

Mid-afternoon _____

Dinner _____

Evening _____

New Foods/Reactions: _____

Stools (amount, number and type): _____

Quick Symptoms Checklist: **Rate Symptoms 0-10**

❏ Headache	❏ Digestive symptoms	Energy level:_____
❏ Joint pain	❏ Abdominal pain	Mood: _____
❏ Muscle pain	❏ Tinnitus	Mental Clarity:_____
❏ Other: _____	❏ Other: _____	Purpose/Hope: _____

Date _____

❑ FCLO/HVBO   ❑ Probiotic   ❑ Detox Bath   ❑ AM Juicing   ❑ Fat
❑ Omega 3/6   ❑ Beet Kvass   ❑ Oil Pull   ❑ PM Juicing   ❑ Stock
❑ Iodine   ❑ Milk Kefir   ❑ Sunbathing   ❑ Movement   ❑ Ferments

Take a Moment:

By failing to prepare, you are preparing to fail. —Benjamin Franklin

What is your plan to be prepared for next year?

_____

_____

_____

_____

Today's Focus: _____

Nutritional Intake:

Breakfast _____

Mid-morning _____

Lunch _____

Mid-afternoon _____

Dinner _____

Evening _____

New Foods/Reactions: _____

Stools (amount, number and type): _____

_____

Quick Symptoms Checklist: **Rate Symptoms 0-10**

❑ Headache   ❑ Digestive symptoms   Energy level:_____
❑ Joint pain   ❑ Abdominal pain   Mood: _____
❑ Muscle pain   ❑ Tinnitus   Mental Clarity:_____
❑ Other: _____   ❑ Other: _____   Purpose/Hope: _____

Date _____

❏ FCLO/HVBO	❏ Probiotic	❏ Detox Bath	❏ AM Juicing	❏ Fat
❏ Omega 3/6	❏ Beet Kvass	❏ Oil Pull	❏ PM Juicing	❏ Stock
❏ Iodine	❏ Milk Kefir	❏ Sunbathing	❏ Movement	❏ Ferments

Take a Moment:

Winter is the time for comfort, for good food and warmth, for the touch of a friendly hand and for a talk beside the fire; It is the time for home.
—Dame Edith Sitwell

What do you love about home?

_____

_____

_____

Today's Focus: _____

Nutritional Intake:

Breakfast _____

Mid-morning_____

Lunch _____

Mid-afternoon _____

Dinner _____

Evening _____

New Foods/Reactions: _____

Stools (amount, number and type): _____

_____

Quick Symptoms Checklist:		**Rate Symptoms 0-10**
❏ Headache	❏ Digestive symptoms	Energy level:_____
❏ Joint pain	❏ Abdominal pain	Mood: _____
❏ Muscle pain	❏ Tinnitus	Mental Clarity: _____
❏ Other: _____	❏ Other: _____	Purpose/Hope: _____

My week overall: 0--10

I would describe my week (in one word) as: _____

Because? _____

General progress:

Advanced to a new stage? Y/N   Current stage?_____

New foods tolerated: _____   Foods removed: _____

Animal fats consumed: _____   Avg. daily amount: _____

# of days stock consumed: _____   Avg. daily amount: _____

Probiotics/fermented foods/cultured dairy:

Probiotic supplement: _____Current dose: _____

Die-off symptoms: Y/N   Describe: _____

_____

Beet Kvass _____   Sour Cream _____

Veggie Medley_____   Yogurt _____

Sauerkraut_____   Kefir_____

Detoxing Progress:

# of detox baths: _____   Ingredients: ACV/Epsom/Baking soda

# of days sunbathed: _____   # of minutes per session:_____ minutes

# of days juiced in am: _____in pm: _____

Ingredients:_____

Overall reactions to detoxing: _____

Symptoms descriptions:

Stools: Daily Y/N   #per day _____   Type(s):_____

Digestion: _____

Mood/energy: _____

Memory/clarity: _____

Sleep/Stress: _____

Typical-for-me symptoms: _____

_____

Date _____

❏ FCLO/HVBO	❏ Probiotic	❏ Detox Bath	❏ AM Juicing	❏ Fat
❏ Omega 3/6	❏ Beet Kvass	❏ Oil Pull	❏ PM Juicing	❏ Stock
❏ Iodine	❏ Milk Kefir	❏ Sunbathing	❏ Movement	❏ Ferments

Take a Moment:

Do not sit still, start moving now. In the beginning you may not go in the direction you want, but as long as you are moving, you are creating alternatives and possibilities. —Rodolfo Costa

Do you stay still until you know exactly what you want?
Can you just start moving today?

_____

_____

Today's Focus: _____

Nutritional Intake:

Breakfast _____

Mid-morning _____

Lunch _____

Mid-afternoon _____

Dinner _____

Evening _____

New Foods/Reactions: _____

Stools (amount, number and type): _____

Quick Symptoms Checklist: **Rate Symptoms 0-10**

❏ Headache	❏ Digestive symptoms	Energy level:_____
❏ Joint pain	❏ Abdominal pain	Mood: _____
❏ Muscle pain	❏ Tinnitus	Mental Clarity:_____
❏ Other: _____	❏ Other: _____	Purpose/Hope: _____

Date _____

❑ FCLO/HVBO	❑ Probiotic	❑ Detox Bath	❑ AM Juicing	❑ Fat
❑ Omega 3/6	❑ Beet Kvass	❑ Oil Pull	❑ PM Juicing	❑ Stock
❑ Iodine	❑ Milk Kefir	❑ Sunbathing	❑ Movement	❑ Ferments

Take a Moment:

> *How much more grievous are the consequences of anger than the causes of it.* —Marcus Aurelius

Has your anger caused more harm than what made you angry?

_____

_____

_____

Today's Focus: _____

Nutritional Intake:

Breakfast _____

Mid-morning _____

Lunch _____

Mid-afternoon _____

Dinner _____

Evening _____

New Foods/Reactions: _____

Stools (amount, number and type): _____

_____

Quick Symptoms Checklist: **Rate Symptoms 0-10**

❑ Headache	❑ Digestive symptoms	Energy level:_____
❑ Joint pain	❑ Abdominal pain	Mood: _____
❑ Muscle pain	❑ Tinnitus	Mental Clarity:_____
❑ Other: _____	❑ Other: _____	Purpose/Hope: _____

Date _____

❏ FCLO/HVBO	❏ Probiotic	❏ Detox Bath	❏ AM Juicing	❏ Fat
❏ Omega 3/6	❏ Beet Kvass	❏ Oil Pull	❏ PM Juicing	❏ Stock
❏ Iodine	❏ Milk Kefir	❏ Sunbathing	❏ Movement	❏ Ferments

Take a Moment:

> *Opportunity may knock only once but temptation leans on the doorbell.* —Oprah Winfrey

Temptations can be persistent. Make a plan to resist temptation (maybe from holiday parties) today.

_____

_____

_____

Today's Focus: _____

Nutritional Intake:

Breakfast _____

Mid-morning _____

Lunch _____

Mid-afternoon _____

Dinner _____

Evening _____

New Foods/Reactions: _____

Stools (amount, number and type): _____

Quick Symptoms Checklist: **Rate Symptoms 0-10**

❏ Headache	❏ Digestive symptoms	Energy level: _____
❏ Joint pain	❏ Abdominal pain	Mood: _____
❏ Muscle pain	❏ Tinnitus	Mental Clarity: _____
❏ Other: _____	❏ Other: _____	Purpose/Hope: _____

Date _____

❑ FCLO/HVBO	❑ Probiotic	❑ Detox Bath	❑ AM Juicing	❑ Fat
❑ Omega 3/6	❑ Beet Kvass	❑ Oil Pull	❑ PM Juicing	❑ Stock
❑ Iodine	❑ Milk Kefir	❑ Sunbathing	❑ Movement	❑ Ferments

Take a Moment:

*Remember that the happiest people are not those getting more,
but those giving more.* —H. Jackson Brown, Jr.

What could you give today?

_____

_____

_____

Today's Focus: _____

Nutritional Intake:

Breakfast _____

Mid-morning _____

Lunch _____

Mid-afternoon _____

Dinner _____

Evening _____

New Foods/Reactions: _____

Stools (amount, number and type): _____

_____

Quick Symptoms Checklist: Rate Symptoms 0-10

❑ Headache	❑ Digestive symptoms	Energy level: _____
❑ Joint pain	❑ Abdominal pain	Mood: _____
❑ Muscle pain	❑ Tinnitus	Mental Clarity: _____
❑ Other: _____	❑ Other: _____	Purpose/Hope: _____

Date _____

❏ FCLO/HVBO	❏ Probiotic	❏ Detox Bath	❏ AM Juicing	❏ Fat
❏ Omega 3/6	❏ Beet Kvass	❏ Oil Pull	❏ PM Juicing	❏ Stock
❏ Iodine	❏ Milk Kefir	❏ Sunbathing	❏ Movement	❏ Ferments

Take a Moment:

Don't cry because it's over, smile because it happened. —Dr. Seuss

Do you usually cry or smile when something is over?

_____

_____

_____

_____

Today's Focus: _____

Nutritional Intake:

Breakfast _____

Mid-morning _____

Lunch _____

Mid-afternoon _____

Dinner _____

Evening _____

New Foods/Reactions: _____

Stools (amount, number and type): _____

Quick Symptoms Checklist:		Rate Symptoms 0-10
❏ Headache	❏ Digestive symptoms	Energy level:_____
❏ Joint pain	❏ Abdominal pain	Mood: _____
❏ Muscle pain	❏ Tinnitus	Mental Clarity: _____
❏ Other: _____	❏ Other: _____	Purpose/Hope: _____

Date _____

❑ FCLO/HVBO	❑ Probiotic	❑ Detox Bath	❑ AM Juicing	❑ Fat
❑ Omega 3/6	❑ Beet Kvass	❑ Oil Pull	❑ PM Juicing	❑ Stock
❑ Iodine	❑ Milk Kefir	❑ Sunbathing	❑ Movement	❑ Ferments

Take a Moment:

Character, the willingness to accept responsibility for one's own life, is the source from which self-respect springs. —Joan Didion

Do you find it easy or difficult to accept responsibility for your own life?

_____

_____

_____

Today's Focus: _____

Nutritional Intake:

Breakfast _____

Mid-morning _____

Lunch _____

Mid-afternoon _____

Dinner _____

Evening _____

New Foods/Reactions: _____

Stools (amount, number and type): _____

Quick Symptoms Checklist: **Rate Symptoms 0-10**

❑ Headache	❑ Digestive symptoms	Energy level: _____
❑ Joint pain	❑ Abdominal pain	Mood: _____
❑ Muscle pain	❑ Tinnitus	Mental Clarity: _____
❑ Other: _____	❑ Other: _____	Purpose/Hope: _____

Date _____

❑ FCLO/HVBO	❑ Probiotic	❑ Detox Bath	❑ AM Juicing	❑ Fat
❑ Omega 3/6	❑ Beet Kvass	❑ Oil Pull	❑ PM Juicing	❑ Stock
❑ Iodine	❑ Milk Kefir	❑ Sunbathing	❑ Movement	❑ Ferments

Take a Moment:

Men succeed when they realize that their failures are the preparation for their victories. —Ralph Waldo Emerson

As you look at the last year, are you ready to accept your failures as preparation for your victories?

_____

_____

_____

Today's Focus: _____

Nutritional Intake:

Breakfast _____

Mid-morning_____

Lunch _____

Mid-afternoon _____

Dinner _____

Evening _____

New Foods/Reactions: _____

Stools (amount, number and type): _____

Quick Symptoms Checklist: **Rate Symptoms 0-10**

❑ Headache	❑ Digestive symptoms	Energy level:_____
❑ Joint pain	❑ Abdominal pain	Mood: _____
❑ Muscle pain	❑ Tinnitus	Mental Clarity:_____
❑ Other: _____	❑ Other: _____	Purpose/Hope:_____

My week overall: 0---10

I would describe my week (in one word) as: _____

Because? _____

General progress:

Advanced to a new stage? Y/N   Current stage?_____

New foods tolerated: _____   Foods removed: _____

Animal fats consumed: _____   Avg. daily amount: _____

# of days stock consumed: _____   Avg. daily amount: _____

Probiotics/fermented foods/cultured dairy:

Probiotic supplement: _____ Current dose: _____

Die-off symptoms: Y/N   Describe: _____

_____

Beet Kvass _____   Sour Cream _____

Veggie Medley_____   Yogurt _____

Sauerkraut_____   Kefir_____

Detoxing Progress:

# of detox baths: _____ Ingredients: ACV/Epsom/Baking soda

# of days sunbathed: _____ # of minutes per session:_____ minutes

# of days juiced in am: _____in pm: _____

Ingredients:_____

Overall reactions to detoxing: _____

Symptoms descriptions:

Stools: Daily Y/N   #per day _____   Type(s):_____

Digestion: _____

Mood/energy: _____

Memory/clarity: _____

Sleep/Stress: _____

Typical-for-me symptoms: _____

_____

Date _____

❏ FCLO/HVBO	❏ Probiotic	❏ Detox Bath	❏ AM Juicing	❏ Fat
❏ Omega 3/6	❏ Beet Kvass	❏ Oil Pull	❏ PM Juicing	❏ Stock
❏ Iodine	❏ Milk Kefir	❏ Sunbathing	❏ Movement	❏ Ferments

Take a Moment:

It's a fine seasoning for joy to think of those we love. —Moliere

Who do you love? Who, when you think of them, brings you joy?

_____

_____

_____

_____

Today's Focus: _____

Nutritional Intake:

Breakfast _____

Mid-morning_____

Lunch _____

Mid-afternoon _____

Dinner _____

Evening _____

New Foods/Reactions: _____

Stools (amount, number and type): _____

_____

Quick Symptoms Checklist: **Rate Symptoms 0-10**

❏ Headache	❏ Digestive symptoms	Energy level:_____
❏ Joint pain	❏ Abdominal pain	Mood: _____
❏ Muscle pain	❏ Tinnitus	Mental Clarity: _____
❏ Other: _____	❏ Other: _____	Purpose/Hope: _____

Date _____

❏ FCLO/HVBO	❏ Probiotic	❏ Detox Bath	❏ AM Juicing	❏ Fat
❏ Omega 3/6	❏ Beet Kvass	❏ Oil Pull	❏ PM Juicing	❏ Stock
❏ Iodine	❏ Milk Kefir	❏ Sunbathing	❏ Movement	❏ Ferments

Take a Moment:

> *I may not have gone where I intended to go, but I think*
> *I have ended up where I needed to be.* —Douglas Adams

Is this where you intended to be? Are you glad you are here, regardless?

_____

_____

_____

Today's Focus: _____

Nutritional Intake:

Breakfast _____

Mid-morning _____

Lunch _____

Mid-afternoon _____

Dinner _____

Evening _____

New Foods/Reactions: _____

Stools (amount, number and type): _____

Quick Symptoms Checklist: **Rate Symptoms 0-10**

❏ Headache	❏ Digestive symptoms	Energy level: _____
❏ Joint pain	❏ Abdominal pain	Mood: _____
❏ Muscle pain	❏ Tinnitus	Mental Clarity: _____
❏ Other: _____	❏ Other: _____	Purpose/Hope: _____

Date _____

❑ FCLO/HVBO	❑ Probiotic	❑ Detox Bath	❑ AM Juicing	❑ Fat
❑ Omega 3/6	❑ Beet Kvass	❑ Oil Pull	❑ PM Juicing	❑ Stock
❑ Iodine	❑ Milk Kefir	❑ Sunbathing	❑ Movement	❑ Ferments

Take a Moment:

Sometimes the best goal you can set is just to get out of bed every day. If you can succeed at this, then other things become possible. —Cynthia Patterson

Getting out of bed, remembering to brush your teeth, these may seem small and silly, but they are important. What small goal can you be okay to set today?

_____

_____

Today's Focus: _____

Nutritional Intake:

Breakfast _____

Mid-morning_____

Lunch _____

Mid-afternoon _____

Dinner _____

Evening _____

New Foods/Reactions: _____

Stools (amount, number and type): _____

Quick Symptoms Checklist:

		Rate Symptoms 0-10
❑ Headache	❑ Digestive symptoms	Energy level:_____
❑ Joint pain	❑ Abdominal pain	Mood: _____
❑ Muscle pain	❑ Tinnitus	Mental Clarity: _____
❑ Other: _____	❑ Other: _____	Purpose/Hope: _____

Date _____

❑ FCLO/HVBO	❑ Probiotic	❑ Detox Bath	❑ AM Juicing	❑ Fat
❑ Omega 3/6	❑ Beet Kvass	❑ Oil Pull	❑ PM Juicing	❑ Stock
❑ Iodine	❑ Milk Kefir	❑ Sunbathing	❑ Movement	❑ Ferments

Take a Moment:

Obstacles are what you see when you take your eyes off of the goal.
—Vince Lombardi

Are you seeing obstacles? Turn them into challenges by looking to your goal.

_____

_____

_____

Today's Focus: _____

Nutritional Intake:

Breakfast _____

Mid-morning_____

Lunch _____

Mid-afternoon _____

Dinner _____

Evening _____

New Foods/Reactions: _____

Stools (amount, number and type): _____

_____

Quick Symptoms Checklist: **Rate Symptoms 0-10**

❑ Headache	❑ Digestive symptoms	Energy level:_____
❑ Joint pain	❑ Abdominal pain	Mood: _____
❑ Muscle pain	❑ Tinnitus	Mental Clarity:_____
❑ Other: _____	❑ Other: _____	Purpose/Hope: _____

Date _____

❑ FCLO/HVBO	❑ Probiotic	❑ Detox Bath	❑ AM Juicing	❑ Fat
❑ Omega 3/6	❑ Beet Kvass	❑ Oil Pull	❑ PM Juicing	❑ Stock
❑ Iodine	❑ Milk Kefir	❑ Sunbathing	❑ Movement	❑ Ferments

Take a Moment:

What is now proved was only once imagined. —William Blake

Think about the last year. What of your imaginings have now been proved?

_____

_____

_____

Today's Focus: _____

Nutritional Intake:

Breakfast _____

Mid-morning_____

Lunch _____

Mid-afternoon _____

Dinner _____

Evening _____

New Foods/Reactions: _____

Stools (amount, number and type): _____

_____

Quick Symptoms Checklist: **Rate Symptoms 0-10**

❑ Headache	❑ Digestive symptoms	Energy level:_____
❑ Joint pain	❑ Abdominal pain	Mood: _____
❑ Muscle pain	❑ Tinnitus	Mental Clarity:_____
❑ Other: _____	❑ Other: _____	Purpose/Hope: _____

Date _____

❑ FCLO/HVBO	❑ Probiotic	❑ Detox Bath	❑ AM Juicing	❑ Fat
❑ Omega 3/6	❑ Beet Kvass	❑ Oil Pull	❑ PM Juicing	❑ Stock
❑ Iodine	❑ Milk Kefir	❑ Sunbathing	❑ Movement	❑ Ferments

Take a Moment:

The secret of getting ahead is getting started. —Mark Twain

What do you want to do? Are you ready to start?

_____

_____

_____

_____

Today's Focus: _____

Nutritional Intake:

Breakfast _____

Mid-morning _____

Lunch _____

Mid-afternoon _____

Dinner _____

Evening _____

New Foods/Reactions: _____

Stools (amount, number and type): _____

Quick Symptoms Checklist:

Rate Symptoms 0-10

❑ Headache	❑ Digestive symptoms	Energy level: _____
❑ Joint pain	❑ Abdominal pain	Mood: _____
❑ Muscle pain	❑ Tinnitus	Mental Clarity: _____
❑ Other: _____	❑ Other: _____	Purpose/Hope: _____

Date _____

❏ FCLO/HVBO	❏ Probiotic	❏ Detox Bath	❏ AM Juicing	❏ Fat
❏ Omega 3/6	❏ Beet Kvass	❏ Oil Pull	❏ PM Juicing	❏ Stock
❏ Iodine	❏ Milk Kefir	❏ Sunbathing	❏ Movement	❏ Ferments

Take a Moment:

> *Hope smiles from the threshold of the year to come,*
> *whispering 'It will be happier.'* —Alfred Lord Tennyson

What are you hoping for next year?

_____

_____

_____

Today's Focus: _____

Nutritional Intake:

Breakfast _____

Mid-morning_____

Lunch _____

Mid-afternoon _____

Dinner _____

Evening _____

New Foods/Reactions: _____

Stools (amount, number and type): _____

Quick Symptoms Checklist: **Rate Symptoms 0-10**

❏ Headache	❏ Digestive symptoms	Energy level:_____
❏ Joint pain	❏ Abdominal pain	Mood: _____
❏ Muscle pain	❏ Tinnitus	Mental Clarity:_____
❏ Other: _____	❏ Other: _____	Purpose/Hope: _____

My week overall: 0--10

I would describe my week (in one word) as: _____

Because? _____

General progress:

Advanced to a new stage? Y/N   Current stage?_____

New foods tolerated: _____   Foods removed: _____

Animal fats consumed: _____   Avg. daily amount: _____

# of days stock consumed: _____   Avg. daily amount: _____

Probiotics/fermented foods/cultured dairy:

Probiotic supplement: _____Current dose: _____

Die-off symptoms: Y/N   Describe: _____

_____

Beet Kvass_____   Sour Cream_____

Veggie Medley_____   Yogurt _____

Sauerkraut_____   Kefir_____

Detoxing Progress:

# of detox baths: _____ Ingredients: ACV/Epsom/Baking soda

# of days sunbathed: _____ # of minutes per session:_____ minutes

# of days juiced in am: _____in pm: _____

Ingredients:_____

Overall reactions to detoxing: _____

Symptoms descriptions:

Stools: Daily Y/N   #per day _____   Type(s):_____

Digestion: _____

Mood/energy: _____

Memory/clarity: _____

Sleep/Stress: _____

Typical-for-me symptoms: _____

_____

Date _____

❏ FCLO/HVBO	❏ Probiotic	❏ Detox Bath	❏ AM Juicing	❏ Fat
❏ Omega 3/6	❏ Beet Kvass	❏ Oil Pull	❏ PM Juicing	❏ Stock
❏ Iodine	❏ Milk Kefir	❏ Sunbathing	❏ Movement	❏ Ferments

Take a Moment:

I give because I know how it feels to want. —Anonymous

Why do you give?

_____

_____

_____

_____

Today's Focus: _____

Nutritional Intake:

Breakfast _____

Mid-morning_____

Lunch _____

Mid-afternoon _____

Dinner _____

Evening _____

New Foods/Reactions: _____

Stools (amount, number and type): _____

Quick Symptoms Checklist: **Rate Symptoms 0-10**

❏ Headache	❏ Digestive symptoms	Energy level:_____
❏ Joint pain	❏ Abdominal pain	Mood: _____
❏ Muscle pain	❏ Tinnitus	Mental Clarity:_____
❏ Other: _____	❏ Other: _____	Purpose/Hope: _____

Date _____

❑ FCLO/HVBO	❑ Probiotic	❑ Detox Bath	❑ AM Juicing	❑ Fat
❑ Omega 3/6	❑ Beet Kvass	❑ Oil Pull	❑ PM Juicing	❑ Stock
❑ Iodine	❑ Milk Kefir	❑ Sunbathing	❑ Movement	❑ Ferments

Take a Moment:

Always give without remembering and always receive without forgetting. —Brian Tracey

What do you remember? What do you forget?

_____

_____

_____

Today's Focus: _____

Nutritional Intake:

Breakfast _____

Mid-morning _____

Lunch _____

Mid-afternoon _____

Dinner _____

Evening _____

New Foods/Reactions: _____

Stools (amount, number and type): _____

Quick Symptoms Checklist: Rate Symptoms 0-10

❑ Headache	❑ Digestive symptoms	Energy level: _____
❑ Joint pain	❑ Abdominal pain	Mood: _____
❑ Muscle pain	❑ Tinnitus	Mental Clarity: _____
❑ Other: _____	❑ Other: _____	Purpose/Hope: _____

Date _____

❏ FCLO/HVBO	❏ Probiotic	❏ Detox Bath	❏ AM Juicing	❏ Fat
❏ Omega 3/6	❏ Beet Kvass	❏ Oil Pull	❏ PM Juicing	❏ Stock
❏ Iodine	❏ Milk Kefir	❏ Sunbathing	❏ Movement	❏ Ferments

Take a Moment:

Change before you have to. —Jack Welch

What is a change you know you should make, but haven't been forced to make yet?

_____

_____

_____

Today's Focus: _____

Nutritional Intake:

Breakfast _____

Mid-morning _____

Lunch _____

Mid-afternoon _____

Dinner _____

Evening _____

New Foods/Reactions: _____

Stools (amount, number and type): _____

Quick Symptoms Checklist: **Rate Symptoms 0-10**

❏ Headache	❏ Digestive symptoms	Energy level:_____
❏ Joint pain	❏ Abdominal pain	Mood: _____
❏ Muscle pain	❏ Tinnitus	Mental Clarity:_____
❏ Other: _____	❏ Other: _____	Purpose/Hope:_____

Date _____

❑ FCLO/HVBO	❑ Probiotic	❑ Detox Bath	❑ AM Juicing	❑ Fat
❑ Omega 3/6	❑ Beet Kvass	❑ Oil Pull	❑ PM Juicing	❑ Stock
❑ Iodine	❑ Milk Kefir	❑ Sunbathing	❑ Movement	❑ Ferments

Take a Moment:

The main dangers in this life are the people who want to change everything or nothing. —Lady Nancy Astor

As you look at next year, how much are you trying to change?

_____

_____

_____

Today's Focus: _____

Nutritional Intake:

Breakfast _____

Mid-morning _____

Lunch _____

Mid-afternoon _____

Dinner _____

Evening _____

New Foods/Reactions: _____

Stools (amount, number and type): _____

Quick Symptoms Checklist: **Rate Symptoms 0-10**

❑ Headache	❑ Digestive symptoms	Energy level:_____
❑ Joint pain	❑ Abdominal pain	Mood: _____
❑ Muscle pain	❑ Tinnitus	Mental Clarity:_____
❑ Other: _____	❑ Other: _____	Purpose/Hope: _____

Date _____

❑ FCLO/HVBO	❑ Probiotic	❑ Detox Bath	❑ AM Juicing	❑ Fat
❑ Omega 3/6	❑ Beet Kvass	❑ Oil Pull	❑ PM Juicing	❑ Stock
❑ Iodine	❑ Milk Kefir	❑ Sunbathing	❑ Movement	❑ Ferments

Take a Moment:

It doesn't matter how many say it cannot be done or how many people have tried it before; it's important to realize that whatever you're doing, it's your first attempt at it. —Wally Amos

Are you considering doing something that others say is impossible?

_____

_____

_____

Today's Focus: _____

Nutritional Intake:

Breakfast _____

Mid-morning _____

Lunch _____

Mid-afternoon _____

Dinner _____

Evening _____

New Foods/Reactions: _____

Stools (amount, number and type): _____

Quick Symptoms Checklist: Rate Symptoms 0-10

❑ Headache	❑ Digestive symptoms	Energy level:_____
❑ Joint pain	❑ Abdominal pain	Mood: _____
❑ Muscle pain	❑ Tinnitus	Mental Clarity: _____
❑ Other: _____	❑ Other: _____	Purpose/Hope: _____

Date _____

❑ FCLO/HVBO	❑ Probiotic	❑ Detox Bath	❑ AM Juicing	❑ Fat
❑ Omega 3/6	❑ Beet Kvass	❑ Oil Pull	❑ PM Juicing	❑ Stock
❑ Iodine	❑ Milk Kefir	❑ Sunbathing	❑ Movement	❑ Ferments

Take a Moment:

The best way to have a good idea is to have lots of ideas. —Linus Pauling

Feeling stuck in something? Brainstorm some ideas, and ask others to help you.

_____

_____

_____

Today's Focus: _____

Nutritional Intake:

Breakfast _____

Mid-morning_____

Lunch _____

Mid-afternoon _____

Dinner _____

Evening _____

New Foods/Reactions: _____

Stools (amount, number and type): _____

_____

Quick Symptoms Checklist: Rate Symptoms 0-10

❑ Headache	❑ Digestive symptoms	Energy level:_____
❑ Joint pain	❑ Abdominal pain	Mood: _____
❑ Muscle pain	❑ Tinnitus	Mental Clarity:_____
❑ Other: _____	❑ Other: _____	Purpose/Hope: _____

Date _____

❏ FCLO/HVBO	❏ Probiotic	❏ Detox Bath	❏ AM Juicing	❏ Fat
❏ Omega 3/6	❏ Beet Kvass	❏ Oil Pull	❏ PM Juicing	❏ Stock
❏ Iodine	❏ Milk Kefir	❏ Sunbathing	❏ Movement	❏ Ferments

Take a Moment:

A mewing cat catches no mice. —Yiddish Proverb

What is something you have been talking about doing?
Plan to do it next year!

_____

_____

_____

Today's Focus: _____

Nutritional Intake:

Breakfast _____

Mid-morning _____

Lunch _____

Mid-afternoon _____

Dinner _____

Evening _____

New Foods/Reactions: _____

Stools (amount, number and type): _____

Quick Symptoms Checklist: **Rate Symptoms 0-10**

❏ Headache	❏ Digestive symptoms	Energy level:_____
❏ Joint pain	❏ Abdominal pain	Mood: _____
❏ Muscle pain	❏ Tinnitus	Mental Clarity:_____
❏ Other: _____	❏ Other: _____	Purpose/Hope: ____

Date _____

- ❑ FCLO/HVBO
- ❑ Omega 3/6
- ❑ Iodine
- ❑ Prociotic
- ❑ Beet Kvass
- ❑ Milk Kefir
- ❑ Detox Bath
- ❑ Oil Pull
- ❑ Sunbathing
- ❑ AM Juicing
- ❑ PM Juicing
- ❑ Movement
- ❑ Fat
- ❑ Stock
- ❑ Ferments

Take a Moment:

The truth of the matter is that you always know the right thing to do. The hard part is doing it. —Norman Schwarzkopf

What is the right thing that you need to do?

_____

_____

_____

Today's Focus: _____

Nutritional Intake:

Breakfast _____

Mid-morning _____

Lunch _____

Mid-afternoon _____

Dinner _____

Evening _____

New Foods/Reactions: _____

Stools (amount, number and type): _____

Quick Symptoms Checklist: **Rate Symptoms 0-10**

- ❑ Headache
- ❑ Joint pain
- ❑ Muscle pain
- ❑ Other: _____

- ❑ Digestive symptoms
- ❑ Abdominal pain
- ❑ Tinnitus
- ❑ Other: _____

Energy level: _____
Moodiness: _____
Mental Clarity: _____
Purpose/Hope: _____

Week-At-A-Glance

My week overall: 0---10

I would describe my week (in one word) as: _____

Because? _____

General progress:

Advanced to a new stage? Y/N   Current stage?_____

New foods tolerated: _____   Foods removed?_____

Animal fats consumed:_____   Avg. daily amount: _____

# of days stock consumed: _____   Avg. daily amount: _____

Probiotics/fermented foods/cultured dairy:

Probiotic supplement: _____Current dose: _____

Die-off symptoms: Y/N   Describe: _____

_____

Beet Kvass _____   Sour Cream_____

Veggie Medley_____   Yogurt _____

Sauerkraut_____   Kefir_____

Detoxing Progress:

# of detox baths: _____ Ingredients: ACV/Epsom/Baking soda

# of days sunbathed: _____ # of minutes per session:_____ minutes

# of days juiced in am: ___ in pm: ___ Ingredients: _____

Overall reactions to detoxing: _____

Symptoms descriptions:

Stools: Daily Y/N   #per day _____   Type(s):_____

Digestion: _____

Mood/energy: _____

Memory/clarity: _____

Sleep/Stress: _____

Typical-for-me symptoms: _____

_____

_____

Final Thoughts

"Finish each day and be done with it. You have done what you could. Some blunders and absurdities no doubt crept in; forget them as soon as you can. Tomorrow is a new day. You shall begin it serenely and with too high a spirit to be encumbered with your old nonsense."

—Ralph Waldo Emerson

Wow! What an accomplishment! Look at what you did these last 365 days! It doesn't matter how many mistakes you made or wrong trails you followed—you did what you could this year, and what you did is amazing!

Celebrate! Tell a friend, journal about it, throw a party, take a day off—however you want to celebrate the profound accomplishment of this past year! You did no small thing; so don't treat it like it was small. You were victorious!

Be proud of what you have done!

And now, tomorrow is coming! When tomorrow comes again you have opportunity again. Opportunity to choose. Opportunity to be grateful. Opportunity to heal. Opportunity to live. Opportunity to do anything.

Your new opportunities await, and you will soon face them. Begin tomorrow calmly but with spirits so high that even you can't get in the way!

Onward!

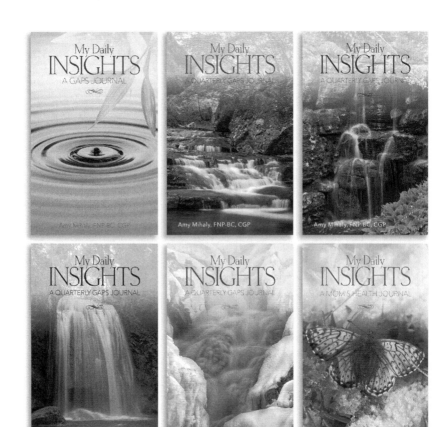

Ready for a new journal?

Visit
www.bewellclinic.net/products
to browse options, and to order.

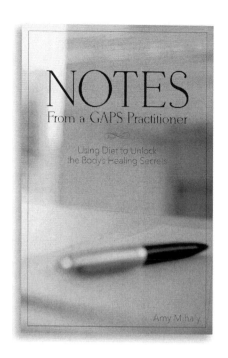

Other Titles by Amy Mihaly

Have you ever been confused about how you should eat, what supplements you should take, or why your body is responding a certain way?

Notes From a GAPS Practitioner: Using Diet to Unlock the Body's Healing Secrets brings understanding and clarity to these confusing topics. Using GAPS principles, this book explains the processes of disease and healing in a way that is easy to understand and apply. Visit www.bewellclinic.net/products for more information, or to order.

Made in the USA
Columbia, SC
21 April 2021